CARB CURFEW™

CARB CURFEW™

CUT THE CARBS AFTER 5PM
AND LOSE FAT FAST!

JOANNA HALL

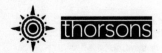

Thorsons
An Imprint of HarperCollins*Publishers*
77–85 Fulham Palace Road
Hammersmith, London W6 8JB

The website address is:
www.thorsonselement.com

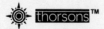 ™

and *Thorsons* are trademarks of
HarperCollins*Publishers* Limited

First published by Thorsons 2003

10 9 8 7 6 5 4 3 2

Joanna Hall's website address is:
www.activeaction.com

Joanna Hall asserts the moral right to
be identified as the author of this work

A catalogue record of this book
is available from the British Library

ISBN 0 00 714742 2

Printed and bound in Great Britain by
Clays Ltd, St Ives plc

CONTENTS

chapter one

Lose Weight – And Still Have a Life!

Most people know to lose weight we have to eat less, but somehow something always seems to get in the way – LIFE! Ask yourself the following questions:

- Do you experience frustration at seeing your weight go up and down on the scales?
- Are you a seasoned dieter who tries every diet available and yet you still don't seem able to shift those extra pounds?
- Do your diet attempts leave you a diet hermit rather than living life to the full?
- Do you want a diet and fitness plan that fits in with your lifestyle – while still achieving your weight and fat-loss goals?

If you have answered yes to any of the above questions then Carb Curfew is for you. The Carb Curfew diet plan shows you the strategies you need to take to lose weight and body fat – and keep it off for good.

Losing weight and body fat is a subject that provokes an array of discussions and fad slimming products and diets. Unfortunately, while some people may claim spectacular results with tablets, potions and 'miracle' foods, the real truth is that long-term weight management requires a little effort and know-how to be able to make it work for you not just for today, but for the future too.

The key to successful weight and body fat loss is simple – it is about good nutrition and how you move your body. The challenge comes when we try to fit a healthy diet into our busy lives – maybe you're running around after your kids all day, or working long hours, or simply leading a jam-packed social life and it feels as though you don't even have time to think about eating well – let alone do it! This is where Carb Curfew steps in. Carb Curfew is adaptable enough to fit in with your life – just the way it is. It allows you to set your own realistic goals, so you don't have to make any radical changes to your lifestyle while you achieve your weight and fat-loss goals.

How Does Carb Curfew Work?

Carb Curfew contains a number of strategies to help you achieve your weight and body fat goals. These nutritional strategies have been tried and tested by my weight-management clients over the last ten years – they have worked for them and they will work for you. The strategies are:

Use the Carb Curfew

By not eating certain carbohydrates after five p.m. you will lose weight and boost your energy levels. It is a strategy that allows you to cut your overall calorie intake and get the right balance of nutrients at the right time of the day. By eating starch with more protein at lunchtime instead of in your evening meal, you will beat your mid-afternoon sugar cravings (the dieter's downfall!) and fuel yourself with energy and brainpower for the rest of the day.

Drink More Water

If you drink less than eight glasses of water a day you may well be chronically dehydrated – this means you will lack energy and your brain will misinterpret this tiredness as a need to eat more food. So by drinking a minimum of two litres of water a day you will fuel yourself with energy, curb your hunger and enhance your nutrient absorption. Stick to the action points in chapter four and you'll be well on the way to a super-hydrated and less hungry body!

Decrease Your Fat Intake

This is not about cutting all fat from your diet – some fat is essential for our health – instead it is about reducing your overall fat intake whilst at the same time increasing the good sources of fat in your diet. By eating 40 grams of the right fats a day you will soon see your own body fat decrease.

Be Consistent

The good news is the best way to lose weight is not to deprive yourself of everything you love, but instead to stick to the 80-20 rule. This means rather than being good 100 per cent of the time, if you can stick to the Carb Curfew diet plan for just 80 per cent of the time you will succeed. Being consistent means you can actually eat a little more and you will still lose weight and body fat and you are not setting yourself up for guilt and 'failure'.

You will also find plenty of recipes in Carb Curfew to help you put the Carb Curfew into practice, as well as lots of suggestions for breakfasts and lunches, and a 14-day eating plan. Everything in this book has been tested by real people with real pressures and their own stories and tips will help you be in control against unwanted excess weight and body fat.

The Key to Long-Term Success

Have you ever beaten yourself up for breaking your new diet that promises to shrink you into your favourite jeans within seven days? Or felt you'd blown your long-term healthy eating plan just because you indulged in a naughty dessert? If you can relate to either of these scenarios then Carb Curfew is definitely for you. It shows you that the key to long-term successful weight management is not to deprive yourself of everything you love or to beat yourself up when you fail – it is about developing and appreciating a balanced and consistent approach to eating, where you only have to be 'good' 80 per cent of the time and you will succeed.

In short, Carb Curfew is about helping you develop strategies that allow you to enjoy the things you want to enjoy, whilst you realize your weight and body fat goals. By following the simple strategies in Carb Curfew, you will have the confidence and know-how to say goodbye to excess weight and body fat – for good.

chapter two

Making Your Diet Work For You

There is no doubt that temptation is thrown at us 24 hours a day, 7 days a week and 365 days a year. Supermarkets re-circulate the smells of their bakery ovens back into the store, ready-prepared foods are becoming more and more convenient and fast food ever more accessible with tempting fare brought right to our front door.

The world we live in today is perpetually stimulating our minds, eyes and taste buds to eat more than we need – to the point where we are almost living in a food-toxic environment. At the same time our society enables us to become less and less active. We are under pressure to achieve more things in one day but the irony is with the wonders of modern technology this results in us expending less physical energy – little wonder then that obesity is rising so dramatically.

Everybody knows that a healthy diet makes sense – not just for today but also for our future health and well-being. But somehow our good intentions never seem to have much staying power. Perhaps it is the thought of a life without a curry or the thought of an existence of carrot sticks and lettuce leaves, but the whole process can seem very unappealing. It's enough to make you reach for the pizza home delivery number and the TV remote control!

But living a healthy life does not mean you have to live a life without chocolate or alcohol. Carb Curfew is about losing weight whilst living the life you wish to live. It is about making small changes matter. It is about knowing how to make dietary choices that work for you. In short, it is about applying a bit of know-how so that you can have your cake and eat it.

Getting Your Diet Right

The first thing we need to look at are the basics of our diet. It is very important to get the fundamentals of our diet right, with the right nutrients in the right balance at the right time. A good diet includes food from each of the four nutrient food groups. These food groups are:

- Carbohydrates
- Proteins
- Fats
- Water

Carbohydrates

Carbohydrates form the backbone of our diet. Fruit, vegetables, simple sugars such as biscuits and cakes, and starches such as potatoes, rice, pasta and bread are all carbohydrates. Carbohydrate-rich foods supply the body with its primary source of fuel – glucose. Glucose is a type of sugar which the body can easily use and transport – when we talk about blood sugars we are actually talking about our blood glucose levels. Glucose can be stored in the muscles as glycogen and is the main source of fuel for our working muscles, the nervous system and brain. We will be talking more about carbohydrates and starch in chapter three.

Proteins

Proteins are essential for tissue repair, maintenance and growth. They are crucial for our health as they make up part of every cell in the body. A regular supply of protein is required in the diet to aid the continual tissue regeneration that occurs in the body. Proteins are made up of smaller units called amino acids. Not all proteins contain all the essential amino acids required by our bodies – this is why if we are vegetarian we need to ensure that we have a variety of protein sources to ensure our bodies are getting a complete range of the necessary proteins. Protein can be divided into two groups: dairy products, which include cheese, yoghurt and eggs; and non-dairy sources, which include meat, fish, pulses and beans. The important role that protein plays in repairing the body means that it is much harder for the body to store excess protein as body fat in the cells.

Dietary Fats

Dietary fats come from a variety of sources. There are various ways of defining fats but one of the simplest is to consider fats as visible and invisible. Visible fats are, as the name suggests, foods that we can see are made of fat. Cheese, butter, oils and creams are examples of visible fats. Invisible fats are foods with a predominant fat content although we may not be aware of it: examples include coconut, avocado and egg yolks. Fats are divided into three groups: saturated, polyunsaturated and monounsaturated. Saturated fats (including unhealthy trans fats) are non-essential fats because they do not play a healthy role in the body and they are associated with an increased risk of heart disease, whereas monounsaturated fats and the omega-3 and omega-6 sources of polyunsaturated fats are essential fats because they have a positive health role to play in the body. Regardless of whether they are essential or non-essential fats they all provide a rich source of energy. See chapter five for more details about dietary fats.

Water

Water is the most overlooked component of our diet – it forms about 60 per cent of our total weight and is involved in every single chemical reaction in the body. If we don't get enough water we are not providing the right environment for our bodies to perform effectively. It is very important to drink at least eight glasses of water a day – it really does impact how you feel and how your body works. See chapter four for more details.

...and Alcohol

While alcohol is not strictly a food group in its own right it does deserve a special mention as it is such a pleasurable part of our daily lives. It is vital however that we understand the role it plays in the body and how it constrains long-term fat loss and weight management. Alcohol does supply us with a source of energy but it is not a nutrient as it is not necessary for life and it is harmful to health when consumed in excess. See page 78 for more about this.

Getting the Balance Right

For your diet to be balanced you need to eat a variety of foods from each food group – the various Carb Curfew diet strategies will go into this in more detail. Carbohydrates should form the backbone of your diet, specifically fruit and vegetables and starchy whole grains. However, don't fall into the trap of eating too many whole-grain starches in the belief that because they are low in fat you can eat more. This is the most common mistake I see with my clients – they may be low in fat but they still contain calories. Proteins should be consumed in a smaller volume and fats should make up the smallest part of your diet.

Most foods contain a variety of protein, fat and carbohydrate, although the combination can vary greatly from one food to another. Hence we tend to define a food by its main food group. If you consume excess calories from any of these food groups – not just fat – you will gain weight and body fat. Whilst some of the nutrients have specific jobs to do, once these jobs have been done any excess calories will simply be stored as fat within our fat cells.

Each of these food groups will provide an energy or calorie value to the body. Carbohydrate and protein provide 4 calories per gram, fat provides 9 calories per gram and alcohol provides 7 calories per gram. So we don't have to be an Einstein to realize that we need to look at the composition of the foods we eat as well as the total number of calories we are consuming if we want to control weight and body fat levels.

Unfortunately, there are no miracle foods to ensure weight loss. It is the whole picture of what we eat that is important for our health, weight and body fat. Carb Curfew will show you that with a little knowledge you can eat whatever you want and still realize your weight and body fat goals.

The Basic Nutrients

CARBOHYDRATES

FRUIT

Typical examples: apples, oranges, pears, grapes, plums

Calories per gram: 4 (fruit and vegetables have a high water content so the calories per weight is kept low)

Function in the body: provides essential minerals and vitamins

When/how much do we need?: minimum 5 portions fruit and vegetables a day (see page 48 for more about this). Spread fruit and vegetable intake throughout day to avoid gastro discomfort

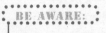
BE AWARE:

most people fall short of quota

VEGETABLES

Typical examples: carrots, kale, onions

Calories per gram: 4 (vegetables, like fruit, have a high water content so the calories per weight is kept low)

Function in the body: provides essential minerals and vitamins

When/how much do we need?: minimum 5 portions fruit and vegetables; spread intake throughout the day

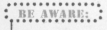

most people fall way short of quota, finding it easier to grab a piece of fruit than hitting the vegetable quota

STARCHES

Typical examples: bread, pasta, rice, potatoes

Calories per gram: 4

Function in the body: good source of fuel for the body to use during the day

When/how much do we need?: 3–4 servings a day. Keep to breakfast and lunch to match energy demands and energy delivery. Avoid in evening meal

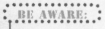

most people mistakenly eat too much when trying to lose weight. Comfort eating of these starchy carbohydrates increases overall calorie intake leading to weight and body fat gain

PROCESSED SUGARS
Typical examples: honey, syrup, jams
Calories per gram: 4
Function in body: provides instant energy into the bloodstream causing the blood sugars to rise and then sharply fall
When/how much do we need?: keep to an absolute minimum. Obtain sugars from natural fruit sources

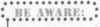

the 4–6 p.m. time zone – the quick sugar-fix craving increases intake of these simple sugars

PROTEIN
Dairy Products
Typical examples: milk, cheese, eggs, yoghurt
Calories per gram: 4
Function in body: repairs vital cells in the body, source of calcium
When/how much do we need?: try to have a serving of protein at each meal

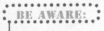

don't eat too much. Be wary of high fat content

Meat, Fish, Pulses
Typical examples: chicken, salmon, cod, beans, nuts
Calories per gram: 4
Function in body: repairs vital cells in the body

When/how much do we need?: try to have a serving at each meal

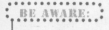

eating protein at lunchtime with an equal amount of starch will boost afternoon concentration powers and leave you feeling more satisfied

FATS
ESSENTIAL FATS
Typical examples: polyunsaturated fat found in vegetable oils and fish oils (in cold water oily fish); monounsaturated fats found in olive oil, rapeseed oil etc.
Calories per gram: 9
Function in body: helps decrease blood cholesterol levels and prevent heart disease
When/how much do we need?: this should form the majority of your fat sources

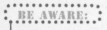

keep visible fats to a minimum and eat 3 servings of oily fish a week

NON-ESSENTIAL FATS
Typical examples: saturated fats such as cheese, cream, lard; trans fats found in margarine, processed foods etc.
Calories per gram: 9
Function in body: potentially increases furring of blood vessels

When/how much do we need?: keep to a minimum

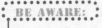

found in a lot of processed foods, especially snacks

WATER
Typical examples: tap, mineral water (either still or sparkling)
Calories per gram: 0
Function in body: vital for all metabolic responses in the body
When/how much do we need?: minimum of 2 litres a day

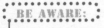

this is one of the most important health investments you can make – it is best to spread your intake throughout the day

ALCOHOL
Typical examples: all wine, liquor, beer
Calories per gram: 7
Function in body: 1–2 units of alcohol per day is thought to have protective effect on the heart
When/how much do we need?: spread consumption of 10 units throughout week

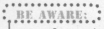

BE AWARE:

if you do overindulge, try to stay up for half an hour before going to bed – it is easier for the liver to work when sitting upright compared to lying down

The Low-Down on Body Fat

So why do we have body fat and how can cutting the carbs help us get rid of it? Whether we like it or not we all have fat in our bodies. Each one of us is born with about 23 billion fat cells and each of these fat cells has the ability to get bigger and bigger, as well as smaller and smaller. A certain amount of fat is important for our bodies as it gives us shape, warmth and insulation – the problem comes when we start to store too much fat in the body from overeating and under activity.

It is inevitable as we get older we are going to lay down more body fat as our body's metabolism changes. To combat this we need to establish a nutritional strategy to minimize body fat gain and improve our overall health. Fat cells do not disappear but the actual amount of fat in the cells can decrease and increase dependent upon how well we eat and how much exercise we take.

How Can We Decrease the Size of our Fat Cells?

Unfortunately, if we are consuming more calories than we are expending our fat cells will get bigger and bigger. Although fat cells do not generally divide and increase in numbers, if we eat excessively and gain a significant amount of weight (40–50 pounds) then our fat cells will get bigger and divide and it is likely that the body fat gained at this time will pose more of a problem to shift. While this may seem depressing it helps explain why sometimes we look at friends and they appear to have dropped the weight effortlessly, while our own efforts seem to require a lot more persistence. Appreciating this will allow you to approach your diet plan with a realistic picture of what you can achieve long-term.

The most effective way to decrease the size of your fat cells is to reduce your weekly intake of calories. Obviously this can be achieved through diet alone, but it is far more effective – and easier – to use a combination of sensible nutrition and physical activity. For fat cells to get smaller we need to create a calorie deficit of 3,500 calories per week. At first sight this figure can appear alarming, however the trick to effective body fat loss is to ensure that the calorie deficit is achieved slowly and consistently. Spreading the 3,500 over seven days means you are aiming for a decrease of 500 calories each day from your normal daily calorie range. If you split these 500 calories between the nutritional strategies in Carb

Curfew and physical activities, the figure becomes a lot more manageable. Incorporating exercise into your routine (whether this involves walking instead of taking the car or fitting in regular sessions at the gym) will go a long way towards helping you achieve your goal.

Ways to Save 500 Calories a Day
- Everyday physical activity: Walk to the post office rather than drive, take the stairs at work, walk up the escalators. Saves you 100 calories.
- Exercise: Power walk for one mile. Saves you 100 calories.
- Nutrition: Operate Carb Curfew in evening meal. Replace a portion of pasta with two portions of extra vegetables. Saves you 200 calories. Replace mid-afternoon snack of 2 slices of bread and jam with an apple. Saves you 100 calories.

Why Do We Gain Weight Faster As We Get Older?

As we get older we actually start to lay down more body fat. This is due to several factors:

1. Metabolic rate

After the age of 30 if we are inactive we actually start to lose muscle mass at a rate of $1/3–1/2$ pound every two years. So if you weighed 10 stone at the age of 20 and you still weigh 10 stone at the age of 50, yet you have gone up two clothes sizes and you do not exercise – quite simply, you have lost muscle mass and gained body fat. As the body fat takes up more space, your clothes become tighter and your clothes size goes up. Muscle is metabolically active, which means that it burns calories. So if we start to lose muscle mass we actually require less calories to do our everyday tasks. Long-term this means we can potentially be consuming the same number of calories at the age of 20 as at the age of 50 but when we are 50 these calories are not burnt off and we are more prone to laying down body fat. This puts our health at risk and we become frustrated with our shape.

2. Hormones

As women start to approach the menopause we enter a stage known as peri menopause – at this time there is a change in our hormones, which may actually encourage our bodies to lay down more body fat.

3. Stress

Yes, stress does make us fat! When we are experiencing long periods of chronic stress such as overwork, or emotional stresses such as a loss of a partner or moving home, there is a change in our metabolism that encourages increased secretion of the hormone cortisol. If this is left unchecked for long periods of time it encourages body fat to be laid down around our midriffs. Research has shown that storing body fat here actually puts us at a greater risk of heart disease.

Whilst this all may seem a little depressing, the best possible course of action you can take is also the most accessible and cheapest – get active! Increasing your level of physical activity has both a positive and immediate impact on your health and ability to control your weight.

Why Do Some People Lose Body Fat Faster Than Others?

Not everyone will lose weight and body fat at the same rate. We are all different, and there are several factors that can affect our rate of weight and body fat loss.

These include:

1. Your existing metabolic rate
2. Your dieting history
3. Your exercise history
4. Your existing eating patterns
5. Your existing activity patterns

1. Your Existing Metabolic Rate

As we have just discussed, our muscle mass starts to decrease as we get older and our metabolic rate tends to slow down, which means we burn fewer calories. Imagine you are 20 years old and you are sitting in a chair, and now imagine you are 50 years old sitting in a chair. Even though you are doing exactly the same everyday activity, if you have not kept up your muscle mass between the ages of 20 and 50 you will be burning less calories sitting still at the age of 50 than sitting still at the age of 20.

2. Your Dieting History

If you are a seasoned dieter and you religiously try every diet on the market and have experienced weight gain/weight loss again and again – long-term it will be harder to lose weight effectively. You may already have experienced this. For example, every January you may have a favourite deprivation diet that gives you great results – well, it did the first couple of times you did it and now you are experiencing frustration as the scales are not giving you the results you want. This is because as the body is continually put through phases of excess and deficit there comes a time when our metabolism may stop working effectively and instead of losing weight we can actually increase the amount of body fat we have. To counteract this you need to stabilize you calorie and fat intake now. Chapter six will show you how to be consistent with your nutrient intake.

3. Your Exercise History

To lose weight and body fat you need to exercise regularly. If you were active when you were younger you will be at an advantage as muscles have a memory – this means that even if you are not exercising now the muscles will be able to respond more effectively and quickly to exercise once you do start. But even if you were not active when you were younger, it is never too late to start. Becoming active now and staying active will help you realize your fat loss goals as well as have an immediate protective effect on your health.

4. Your Existing Eating Patterns

Quite simply, the more erratic our eating patterns the harder it is to lose weight, and the longer you have had erratic eating patterns the more frustration you are likely to experience trying to lose weight. The body actually balances itself out over seven to eight days; however, in those seven to eight days if you have overeaten one day and then starved yourself the next in an attempt to make up for the excesses, the body will rebel and you will not lose weight and body fat.

To lose body fat, and for us to actually see a difference in the shape of our bodies, we need to eat a healthy and balanced diet and be consistent about it. Start now – apply the Carb Curfew, cut your intake of fat and be consistent.

5. Your Existing Activity Patterns

If you are reading this and are frustrated because you already exercise – or consider yourself to have a pretty active daily routine – and are still not losing weight, this may be a result of the following:

- You do not have enough variety in your exercise programme and your body has become complacent at always doing the same thing.

- The activities that are part of your daily routine are not putting your body under enough physiological strain to increase your fitness.

If you are reading this thinking it's about time I became more active – then what are you waiting for?

Where Do We Store Our Body Fat?

Have you ever wondered why some of us seem to store all our body fat on our hips and thighs and some of us tend to have long lean arms and legs but store more of our body fat around our midriffs? This distribution of fat is associated directly to two main hormones in the body. These hormones, lipoprotein lipase LPL and hormone sensitive lipase HSL, directly affect whether we store fat or encourage it to be distributed in the blood and then burnt off. LPL tends to encourage fat storage and HSL tends to encourage fat to be burnt off. The amount of LPL and HSL we have tends to vary between men and women, individuals and areas of the body.

Men tend to have more LPL in the belly and less HSL in the lower hip area. This creates the more pronounced apple shape we see in overweight men, with more body fat distributed around the belly. Women tend to have more LPL in the hips and back of the arms and less HSL in the upper body. This classically creates more of our traditional pear shape. When women lose weight we generally still have more LPL in the hips so still have a pear shape.

So the challenge for us is to try and create more HSL and one of the best ways to do this is with exercise. Weight-bearing aerobic exercise such as brisk walking, jogging and aerobics is the best form of exercise to choose. Swimming, even though it is an aerobic activity, has shown to be less effective for weight loss as it is non-weight bearing so it is not so effective in burning off calories. In addition, swimming increases LPL, which has the effect of decreasing our core temperature, which in turn can stimulate us to eat more.

Carb Curfew will help you reduce your weight and body fat and boost your confidence to put you in control long-term. It is important to understand however that due to your own individual makeup your body will have an optimum shape it naturally wants to be.

Why Is Measuring Body Fat Important?

When we stand on weighing scales we are actually measuring our total body weight, which is made up of muscle tissue (also known as muscle mass or fat-free mass) and fat tissue (also known as fat mass). Muscle is denser than body fat, so if you took a pound of muscle and you took a pound of fat, the pound of fat would take up a lot more space. It is the amount of fat that we have in our bodies that actually affects our body shape and health. The reading we receive from traditional bathroom scales tells us what the total amount of our body weight is – body fat and muscle (and other tissue such as bone) – but it does not tell us how much fat we actually have. It is this excess body fat that is associated with heart disease, high blood pressure, diabetes and certain types of cancer. By measuring our body fat not only are we monitoring how much of our weight is actually fat but it also gives us an indicator of our health status. Monitoring our percentage body fat actually allows us to impact our health by ensuring we lose body fat as opposed to muscle mass.

Studies have shown that with very low calorie diets, the body will actually lose muscle mass and keep hold of body fat. This means that with some 'diets' you may actually increase the amount of body fat you have!

How Can I Measure How Much Body Fat I Have?

Body fat can be measured in a number of ways. One method is with skin-fold calipers. The skin folds are generally taken at four sites around the body.

A more convenient and accurate method to measure in your own home however is with body fat monitors. Constructed as a set of bathroom weighing scales, by entering your height and sex and standing on the scales, a safe technique known as bioelectrical impedance analysis will determine your percentage body fat. Replacing bathroom scales with body fat monitors will give a true idea of what is happening inside you – this way you get to see a complete picture of your total body weight, muscle mass and fat mass. Body fat monitors are now available from a wide range of outlets.

How Much Body Fat Should We Have?

We all need to have body fat. Too little and we run the risk of decreased fertility and the onset of amenorrhea, a condition where the female periods stop. Too much body fat is associated with an increased risk of heart disease, hypertension, diabetes and some cancers. So what exactly are the healthy ranges? The figures shown below are broadly accepted as the ideal percentages for body fat.

Males
Age 18–39:   8%–20%
Age 40–59:   11%–22%
Age 60+:   13%–25%

Females
Age 18–39:   21%–33%
Age 40–59:   23%–34%
Age 60+:   24%–36%
Source: European Congress of Obesity, 1999

What Fat-Loss Target Should We Aim For?

Changing body fat does take time but the benefits you see will be long-term. A two to four per cent decrease in body fat over a ten-week period is a sensible and realistic target. Although this may not sound a lot, in real terms this will represent a two to four per cent decrease in the amount of fat your body is actually carrying with you day in and day out.

Recording Your Progress

It is good to keep a record of how much body fat you are losing each week so you can see how much progress you are making. Here is what you do:

- Weigh yourself and establish your percentage body fat (either with a body fat monitor or with skin-fold calipers), or if this is not possible then record your weight and tape measurements only.
- Using a tape measure, establish your waist measurement (measure around narrowest part of midriff), your belly button measurement (measure around midriff over belly button) and hip measurement.
- Record these measurements at the same time each week.

Factors Determining Your Success

Your Willpower

The strength of your willpower is an important factor in how successful you will be at realizing your weight and body fat goals. Generally an individual's willpower is at its weakest towards the end of the day – perhaps we feel tired or our blood sugars are low. This means that we tend to have less control of our actions at this time and are more likely to overeat or eat all the inappropriate foods. If you are constantly tired and struggling with your weight, you may well be building up extra calories at the end of the day that do not get burnt off. Here are a few questions for you to think about:

1. When am I most physically active?
   - between 7 a.m. to 6 p.m.
   - after 6 p.m. to bedtime
2. When do I consume the majority of my food?
   - between 7 a.m. to 6 p.m.
   - after 6 p.m. to bedtime
3. When is my willpower at its strongest?
   - first thing in the morning
   - midday
   - mid-afternoon
   - evening

Invariably what happens is there is a mismatch between when we need to receive energy from our food and when we are expending energy through our everyday activities. Generally we expend most energy between 7 a.m. in the morning and 6 p.m. in the evening. However, we actually receive the vast majority of our energy from food after 6 p.m. when we are less active. While some studies suggest that it makes no difference whether your calories from food are consumed during the day or all at night, what these studies fail to take into account is our personal willpower. At the end of the day when we are tired, especially when we have not eaten much during the day, willpower will be low and we will be much more likely to overeat. This means long-term there is a situation where at the end of each day there is actually a build up of excess calories which we are not burning off prior to going to bed – and these calories are being laid down in the fat cells as additional body fat. Carb Curfew will show you how to make the right food choices at the right time of the day, so you receive energy when you need it and you don't end up with a build up of excess calories before you go to bed.

Your Attitude to Food

What we were introduced to as a child defines our relationship with food in later life. If you ate a lot of sugar and sweet things as you were growing up and your diet did not include a variety of tastes, it is likely you now crave calorie-dense sweet foods rather than savoury foods. Maybe your mother used to say to you, 'You must finish everything on your plate', and now you always finish everything on your plate thinking it is rude to leave even a morsel. Or alternatively you had a mother who was always on a diet and never ate the same food as the rest of the family. Our mums are great but we need to be aware of how their attitude to food influences our attitude to food later in life. These attitudes have had a long time to become ingrained and they will take a long time to diminish. Carb Curfew will help you re-evaluate your relationship with food, showing you how to draw up a sensible eating plan that will help you realize your weight and body fat goals, as well as providing a positive message for your children.

Your Motivation

What is your motivation to lose weight? Is it to squeeze into that little black dress for a certain event or is it about looking better for a significant A.N. Other? Whatever your motivation you need to identify it and shift it from an external motivation such as an important event to an internal one such as wanting to feel more in control of your eating habits, have more energy and feel better about yourself. All of which translates into a strategy that you can incorporate and build on to achieve your long-term weight and body fat goals. Think about this: what we weigh in seven years will not be determined by what we do for the next seven minutes, seven hours or the next seven days but how well we eat for the next seven years. Following an action plan that you can keep to will be crucial – Carb Curfew will show you how to do this. Seeing results is a huge motivation and with a little effort that motivation can be your driving force.

Your Friends

Early on in your efforts you need to establish who are going to be saboteurs and supporters of your aims. Within your circle of friends and family there will be individuals who will encourage you and help you with your efforts. It is also likely there will be individuals who either intentionally or unintentionally try to hinder you – this may be because your effort and seeing you look and feel better makes them feel less comfortable or they are just genuinely unaware of their intentions. Identifying who are your diet friends and foes will help you apply the Carb Curfew strategies more effectively and successfully.

Personalizing the Diet

As you work through the book you will be able build up your own personal plan, using the nutritional strategies to help you realize your goals. It is important to understand that there is no one diet that works for everyone; instead Carb Curfew contains strategies that can accommodate many different lifestyles. As you read through think about the best method of fitting the strategies into your life, for instance which lunches are most appropriate if you work in an office, how you can reach your water intake goal while running after the kids all day, or how you can use the Carb Curfew concept to continue enjoying your busy social life.

A Final Word

So, remember, Carb Curfew is about losing weight whilst still living the life you wish to live. Yes, it does require a little bit of effort but you don't have to make any big sacrifices or radical changes to your lifestyle to get the results you want – all you need to do is apply the four strategies outlined on pages 3–4 and you will achieve your weight and fat-loss goals not just for now, but for the future too.

Take Action

- Write a list of the main obstacles to you achieving your fat-loss goals – try to be as specific as possible, for example, mid-morning coffee break with work colleagues or tea time with the kids when you are starving yourself.
- Make a commitment today to make one small change in your daily activities that you will keep up for the next six weeks. For example, say no to coffee in your mid-morning break and have a cup of herbal tea instead. Remember, every small change you make will take you one step further towards achieving your fat-loss goals.

chapter three

The Carb Curfew

We all know we have to steer clear of a diet that contains too much fat and we feel proud of ourselves if we have said no to chocolate or ice-cream. So why are we still struggling with our weight and body fat? These days one of the most common reasons for our weight-loss frustrations is that we have come to rely on low-fat starches and we are lulled into a false sense of low-fat security, thinking we can eat more of these foods. A high consumption of starch however can provide more calories than we need. If we are unable to burn off these calories they become stored as fat, all of which leads to the scales and belt notches not moving in the direction we want.

So the first part of the Carb Curfew strategy is to operate a Carb Curfew. In this chapter you'll learn all about the role of starch and its impact on the body and how to:

⊚ Use the Carb Curfew – no starches after 5 p.m.
⊚ Adapt your meals to make sure you get the right range of nutrients and don't eat too much starch.
⊚ Make good food choices when you are faced with a situation where there is starch on the menu and you are not allowed to eat it.

Carb Curfew Essentials

The two keys to making carbohydrates work for you are:

1. Operate the Carb Curfew to decrease total calorie intake.
2. Consume five portions of fruit and vegetables a day.

What is the Carb Curfew?

As we discussed in chapter two starch, processed sugars and fruit and vegetables are all carbohydrates. The starch foods are potatoes, bread, rice, pasta and cereals, all of which provide a good source of fuel for the body to use during the day.

The Carb Curfew means you can eat starch at breakfast, lunch and in your mid-afternoon snack but you are not allowed to eat it after 5 p.m. The evening meal now comprises of protein, fruit and vegetables, low-fat dairy products and essential fats. It is a strategy that allows you to get the right balance of calories and nutrients at the right time in the day. At first this may seem a little difficult to apply but you will soon feel the huge benefits in your energy levels and you'll certainly appreciate the change in your body shape as you become less bloated.

The Carb Curfew however is not just about saying no to starches after 5 p.m. – it is about getting the right balance of your overall intake of starches and nutrients throughout the day. For example you may be consuming too many calories from starch foods which are contributing to your body fat, so once you reduce the amount of starch you eat you will lose weight and body fat. Also, you will be more in control of your energy levels as you will be eating the right amount of starch at the right time for optimum energy. We will talk more about this later in the chapter.

Are You a Carb Comfort-Eater?

Answer the following questions to find out if you are prone to overeating on comfort starches such as bread, pasta, rice and potatoes.

- Do you tend to snack on bread and comfort carbohydrates such as cakes and chocolate?
- Do you munch bread with each meal?
- Do you feel lethargic in the afternoons?
- Do you eat most of your calories at the end of your day?
- Do you crave carbohydrates?
- Do you experience swings in your energy and mood?
- Do you find it difficult to stop eating comfort starches like biscuits, bread and pasta?

If you answered yes to most of these questions you are sensitive to comfort carbohydrates, specifically the comfort foods that are starch-based. You probably have a tendency to eat more of these foods than is appropriate and this causes you to feel lethargic and out of control. As well as operating the Carb Curfew, you need to use the starch-free zone (see page 61) when faced with an excess starch situation.

If your answers were mainly negative, you are less prone to overindulging on carbohydrates. If you experience problems with your weight it may be due to excess calories consumed through carbohydrates or an imbalance in your nutrient intake. Introduce the Carb Curfew as a tool to control calorie intake.

Watch Those Calories!

I developed the Carb Curfew concept as a nutritional diet tool when I realized a number of my weight management clients were experiencing initial weight and body fat loss but then they were reaching a plateau with their weight loss and their efforts seemed to go no further. This seemed to be a recurring theme, not just with my clients but also with other people's initial weight-loss success stories.

My clients were all very efficient at decreasing the overall fat in their diets, but because their focus was on fat their attention slipped from their carbohydrate intake – specifically bread, pasta, rice, potatoes and cereal were all being over-consumed and often in the evening as opposed to during the day when our body may burn these nutrients more effectively. A typical daily food intake looked something like this:

Breakfast: cereal with skimmed milk and banana
Lunch: large jacket potato with sweetcorn, one banana
Snack: chunk of bread with fruit jam
Dinner: pasta with homemade tomato sauce, brown bread roll

Now at first glance this seems to be a pretty healthy diet and to a certain extent it is, however what it lacks is essential fats, a minimum of five portions of fruit and vegetables, protein and suitable portion sizes. The classic mistake is that too many calories were being consumed. So while fat intake was decreased and in fact very low, the consumption of calories through starches was increasing.

Total calorie intake does count. So while we may be very good at reducing the amount of fat in our diet, if the total number of calories consumed is higher than the amount of calories being burnt off through exercise and activity, then weight gain can actually occur regardless that the source of calories were 'fat-free'.

Have a look at the table below to see the calorie content of some typical starch foods – this will help you to see how excess calories from starch might be contributing to your body fat.

Calorie Content of Starch Foods

Food	Calorie Value
1 large slice wholemeal bread	100
pasta (100g dry weight)	405
rice (100g dry weight)	400
1 jacket potato (200g raw weight)	160
1 bagel	225
1 croissant	295
1 large pitta	180
1 hot cross bun	190

bowl of bran flakes (40g)	147
1 naan bread	450
4 roast potatoes (200g)	340
1 burger bun	140
slice of focaccia bread	160
1 crumpet	80

What Are the Benefits of Using the Carb Curfew?

As I explained at the beginning of the chapter, you can eat starch in moderation at breakfast, lunch and in your mid-afternoon snack but you cannot eat it in your evening meal. By operating the Carb Curfew you will:

◎ Help decrease your overall calorie intake.
◎ Help decrease your overall starch intake. Excess starch stimulates the production of serotonin in the brain, which can make us feel more sluggish. This in turn directly stimulates us to reach for the instant high of a sugar fix such as chocolate, sugary sweet cakes, biscuits and processed snacks.
◎ Beat your sugar cravings. Eating the right amounts of protein and starch at lunchtime will fuel you with energy and brainpower all afternoon.

Why Does the Carb Curfew Work?

The Carb Curfew works because:

1. By eating your starch at breakfast and lunch, it means you consume more energy-providing nutrients during the day. This will give you more physical and mental energy to meet the daily demands and pleasures of life.
2. It allows you to have a lighter meal in the evening based on protein and fruit and vegetables. This helps you achieve a healthier balance of nutrients, as without the presence of bread, pasta, rice,

grains and potatoes you will really need to fill up on fruit and vegetables.

3. Eating less in the evening will make you hungry for a lovely healthy breakfast – this will fuel you with energy right through the day.

The Low-Down on Carbohydrates

Should We Eat Carbohydrates?

Yes, carbohydrates form the backbone of our diet. Fruit and vegetables should be eaten at each meal; starches can be eaten at breakfast and lunch but not in your evening meal, and processed sugars should be kept to an absolute minimum. It is important to remember that the different types of carbohydrates are treated by the body in different ways. The trick to successful weight and body fat loss is to make sure you are eating the right carbohydrates at the right time of the day, so your body receives the right type of carbohydrate when it needs it. This will help you achieve and maintain your weight and body fat goals, you will have more energy during the day, and most importantly, you will minimize your hunger pangs.

To help you understand how the Carb Curfew works, the following summary shows you when to eat what carbohydrate foods for optimum energy and weight loss.

Carbohydrates

Starches

Food examples: all breads, pasta, rice, potatoes, sweet potatoes, cereal, oats, bulgur wheat, millet
When to eat: breakfast, lunch and afternoon snack – you are not allowed to consume in mid-morning snack or after 5 p.m.

Fruit

Food examples: apples, nectarines, melons, raspberries
When to eat: all meals and snacks, especially in evening meal

Vegetables

Food examples: peppers, broccoli, carrots, mushrooms
When to eat: all meals and snacks, especially in evening meal

Processed sugars

Food examples: sweets, chocolates, cakes, biscuits
When to eat: minimal consumption

What is the Glycaemic Index?

Traditionally carbohydrate foods, which provide the main fuel base for our bodies, are classified as simple or complex carbohydrates. Simple carbohydrates such as sugars, some fruits, cakes and biscuits provide a quick increase in blood glucose levels whilst complex carbohydrates such as brown rice, porridge oats and wholegrains raise blood glucose at a slower rate and keep blood glucose levels more stable for longer. The rate at which our blood sugars change with eating different types of carbohydrates is called the glycaemic index (GI).

The concept of GI carbohydrates is fairly new and is particularly recommended for individuals who may be sensitive to swings in energy. The text below illustrates the GI of some common carbohydrate foods. Pure sugar receives a value of 100, and other sugary foods and starches are compared to that. Later in the chapter, to help you optimize your energy levels, we'll look at when it is best to eat which GI carbohydrates.

Glycaemic Index Carbohydrates

Food and its GI rating

sugar	100
carrots, cornflakes, honey, parsnips, potatoes	80–90
wholewheat bread, white rice	70–79
bananas, white bread, raisins, brown rice	60–69
porridge oats, frozen peas, pasta, sweet potatoes	50–59
oranges, orange juice, dried peas, apples, fructose	below 50

Is it Okay to Grab a Quick Sugar Fix?

Sugar gives us an instant release of energy, which is then followed by an energy low. When we consume a large concentrated form of sugar, such as a slice of chocolate cake or a commercially made muffin, the hormone insulin reacts to the elevated blood glucose levels and transfers the sugar from the blood into the cells. This response is so effective that the body can decrease the blood sugar levels very effectively. This in turn creates a feeling of further tiredness, lack of energy and increased appetite about 90 minutes after you had your first sugar fix. So while sugar has a role to play in the diet, its ability to provide a quick instant energy boost is short-lived and can create a roller-coaster of high and low blood sugar levels, which sends us craving more sugar as well as for some of us causing depression and continued fatigue. So instead of relying on sugar from sweets we need to rely more on the natural sources of sugars from fruit and vegetables to stabilize our blood sugar levels.

How Much Fruit and Vegetables Should We Eat?

The World Health Organization recommends we eat at least five portions of fruit and vegetables a day. But what exactly is one portion? Unfortunately the slice of tomato in our sandwich does not equal a portion. And sorry, potatoes do not count, as they are a starch.

Here are some examples of the amount of fruit and vegetables in one portion:

- ◎ apple, orange or banana – 1 fruit
- ◎ very large fruit e.g. melon, pineapple – 1 large slice
- ◎ small fruits e.g. plums, kiwi, satsuma – 2 fruit
- ◎ raspberries, strawberries, grapes – 1 cup
- ◎ fresh fruit salad, stewed or canned – 1–1¹/2 cups
- ◎ dried fruit – 1 cup
- ◎ fruit juice – 1 glass (150ml)
- ◎ vegetables, raw, cooked, frozen or canned – 1 cup
- ◎ salad – 1 dessert bowl

Count up what you are eating now – if it is less than five portions a day, add in one more and gradually build up to five.

What About Fibre?

Fibre is the indigestible portion of carbohydrate. There are two types of fibre: soluble fibre found mainly in fruits, vegetables and in some grains, particularly oats, and insoluble fibre found mainly in the bran portion of cereal grains. Research has shown that a diet rich in soluble fibre is associated with a reduced risk of developing heart disease and diabetes, while a diet rich in insoluble fibre will help reduce cholesterol levels and is beneficial for bowel movement. No single food supplies all the soluble and insoluble fibre needed for health, so a wide variety of min-imally processed, high-fibre foods as included in the Carb Curfew plan are recommended. Studies linking fibre to a reduced risk of disease have investigated naturally occurring fibre-rich foods such as vegetables, fruits, beans and whole-grains. Be wary of commercialized fibre-based products such as bran muffins as these are often high in fat, sugar or salt.

Eating for Energy

The key to the Carb Curfew is to keep your energy levels up by making sure you eat the right type of carbo-hydrate at the right time of day. The following guidelines, in conjunction with the eating plans and recipes at the end of the book, will help you put the Carb Curfew into practice.

When to Eat Your Carbohydrates

Foods with a High Glycaemic Index Rating
Food examples: bread, bagels, pastry, cornflakes, pota-toes, rice, parsnips, raisins, bananas, chocolate, sweet and semi-sweet biscuits
When to eat: breakfast, lunch, after an exercise session. Do not eat in your evening meal. Operate the Carb Curfew

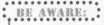

consuming high GI foods at breakfast can leave you feeling hungry later in the morning, so consume with some protein to offset fast release of sugars, e.g. wholemeal toast with boiled egg or have a glass of milk with your toast

Foods with a Moderate Glycaemic Index
Food examples: pasta, porridge oats, noodles, oatmeal biscuits, sweet potatoes, grapes
When to eat: breakfast, lunch, after an exercise session

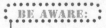

if you are prone to lapses of energy mid-morning, choose a moderate GI carbohydrate for breakfast. Consume with some protein to provide slow release of energy during the day. Porridge and oatmeal are your best choice at breakfast

Foods with a Low Glycaemic Index Rating
Food examples: most fruit and vegetables
When to eat: breakfast, lunch, evening meal

BE AWARE:

consume with protein sources for evening meal

When to Eat Your Starches

Breakfast
Choose: a high or moderate GI source of starch with a piece of fruit
Food example: porridge made with skimmed milk, served with a handful of raisins and half a banana

Mid-morning Snack
Choose: no starch, only fruit or vegetables
Food example: peach, pear, vegetable crudité

Lunch
Choose: a high or moderate GI source of starch with a serving of protein
Food example: open tuna salad sandwich

Mid-afternoon Snack
Choose: a moderate source of starch (though a piece of fruit or yoghurt or smoothie is a better choice as this will hydrate the body)
Food example: slice of rye bread with fruit spread

Evening Meal
Choose: Carb Curfew so no bread, pasta, rice, potatoes, cereal after 5 p.m.
Eat protein with vegetables and fruit

Food example: grilled steak with mushrooms, onions and peppers sautéed in a teaspoon of olive oil, served with large salad made with rocket, spinach, tomatoes, peppers, carrots and watercress

Starting The Day Right

You can optimize your energy and put yourself in the best possible position to achieve your weight and body fat goals by starting your day with the right type of breakfast.

Breakfast

Starting your day with a healthy breakfast is important as it refuels your body and provides you with energy right through the day. However, you need to make sure you get the right type of breakfast to minimize hunger pangs mid-morning. Here are some examples of breakfasts which will boost your energy first thing in the morning, whilst keeping your calorie intake down.

Top Breakfasts

The list below gives examples of breakfasts which are low in fat and nutrient-dense. They are in no particular order.

- Porridge with Raspberries: 30g of porridge oats made with skimmed milk. Serve with a handful of raspberries.
- Boiled Egg with a slice of Wholemeal Toast: Serve with a glass of orange juice.
- Summer Fruit Salad: Large bowl of strawberries, honeydew melon and nectarines. Serve with a small handful of rolled oats and 150g pot of plain low-fat yoghurt.
- Bran Cereal with Apricots and Sultanas: Mix together 30g bran cereal, 2 dried apricots and 15g sultanas and add 1/4 pint skimmed milk. Serve with a small glass of grapefruit juice.
- Banana Smoothie: 1 ripe banana (frozen), 250ml semi-skimmed milk, 1 tablespoon wheatgerm, 4 strawberries. Blend and go.
- Raisin Toast with Sliced Plum: Spread 2 slices raisin toast with quark and top with sliced plum.
- Swiss Muesli: Soak 30g porridge oats overnight with enough water to cover. Serve with skimmed milk or low-fat live bio yoghurt and a pinch of nutmeg, sultanas and grated apple.
- Wholemeal Toast with Cottage Cheese and Marmite: Spread 2 slices of wholemeal toast with cottage cheese and marmite or yeast spread.
- Poached Egg with Wholemeal Toast: Add a dash of Worcestershire sauce for seasoning and serve with 2 slices of wholegrain toast and 1/2 grilled tomato.

◎ Citrus Medley and Open Bacon Sarnie: Segment
$1/2$ orange grapefruit and $1/2$ pink grapefruit – and
season with ground cinnamon. Serve with one slice
of toasted soda bread with two lean grilled bacon
rashers.

You will find further breakfast ideas in the 14-Day Carb
Control Diet chapter.

Getting it Right in the Middle of the Day

Eating the right foods at lunchtime will fuel you with
energy for the afternoon, help you avoid those mid-
afternoon sugar pangs and help stabilize your calorie
intake through the day. To make this work for you, you
need to eat an equal amount of protein and starch in your
midday meal.

Why Do I Need Protein at Lunchtime?

It is really important to eat protein at lunchtime as it
increases the release of the hormone-like substance
dopamine in our body. As I mentioned earlier, this is a
brain transmitter which helps us to feel more alert,
improves our concentration and helps regulate moods.
Often we feel lethargic after lunch – this may be because

we consume the wrong balance of nutrients in our mid-day meal. If we eat too much starch at lunchtime it increases the amount of serotonin in the brain, which may make us feel more lethargic. You need to eat protein with starch at lunchtime and preferably in the ratio of one portion of starch to one portion of protein. This means instead of having a sandwich with two pieces of bread and a ham filling (this gives a food ratio of two starch to one protein), you eat an open ham sandwich with one piece of bread (this gives a food ratio of one starch to one protein). Not only does this help to give you a better balance of nutrients, it will also save you calories.

What is a Portion Size?

Have a look at the following list to find out how much a portion of starch and protein is. Knowing exactly how much starch and protein we are eating will help us get the food ratio right at lunchtime.

You can also visually estimate portion size for convenience. The general rule is that a portion of starch looks roughly the same size as a portion of protein. This means, for example, if you are having a jacket potato you will add a portion of cottage cheese roughly the same size as the potato. Or if you are making an open sandwich you will add a layer of protein, such as tuna or chicken, the same thickness as the slice of bread.

One Portion of Starch Equals:

1 slice regular bread

2 slices 'extra thin' or 'diet' bread

1/2 English muffin

1/2 hotdog or hamburger bun

1 small dinner roll

1/2 cup starchy vegetables

1/2 cup mashed potato or 1 small baked potato

1/2 cup cooked cereal, pasta or rice

1 x 6-inch tortilla

30g cold cereal

4–6 crackers

3 cups air-popped popcorn

2 rice cakes or 5 mini-cakes

One Portion of Protein Equals:

Dairy

1 cup of skimmed milk

1/4 cup semi-skimmed milk

3/4 cup fruit-flavoured yoghurt

1 cup non-fat yoghurt

1/2 cup low-fat yoghurt

42–56g low-fat cheese

30g natural cheese

1/2 cup cottage cheese

Meat, Fish, Poultry and Eggs
84g cooked lean meat, fish or poultry
1/2 cup cooked beans
1 medium egg

And Don't Forget About Pulses ...

Pulses such as kidney, cannellini and flageolet beans are important ingredients in the Carb Curfew diet. As I mentioned earlier, we define foods by their main food group – so although pulses are defined as proteins they also have a carbohydrate content. Pulses score a low GI index rating, which means that they produce a small rise in blood sugar levels, which helps us to stabilize energy levels and mood swings. Pulses are a great addition to both our midday and evening meal.

Top Lunches

The following list shows you how to obtain the right ratio of starch and protein at lunchtime. (Note: portion size does matter!)

- Open Sandwich: 1 slice pumpernickel bread, 100g smoked salmon, 1 tablespoon low-fat yoghurt and a garnish of cod roe. Serve with a large spinach salad.
- Jacket Potato with Cottage Cheese: 200g potato with 150g reduced-fat cottage cheese. Serve with side salad.

- Brown Rice, Kidney Bean and Pea Salad: 1 cup of cooked brown rice with 1/2 cup of kidney beans and peas. Dress in balsamic vinegar dressing made with 1/2 teaspoon olive oil.
- Boiled Egg: Serve with 3 ryvitas and 2 tomatoes.
- Vegetable Soup with Beans: 500ml carton of non-cream based vegetable soup with 1/2 cup of kidney beans or quinoa.
- Chargrilled Chicken Wrap: Soft flour tortilla filled with grilled, poached or roast chicken breast (no skin), sliced tomato, 2 slices of avocado, 1/2 tablespoon natural yoghurt and sprinkled with fresh coriander.
- Sushi: Mixed medium sushi box (250g). Serve with a small glass of orange juice.
- BLT Pitta: Wholemeal pitta bread filled with salad, 25g grilled lean back bacon (all visible fat removed), small boiled egg and a sliced tomato.
- Soup with Tofu: 500ml carton of commercial or home-made non-cream based vegetable soup with 100g cubed tofu.
- Pasta Salad: 100g cooked pasta shapes mixed with 150g pot of low-fat cottage cheese, chopped tomato and fresh basil. Season with salt and pepper.

You will find further ideas for your midday meal in the Carb Curfew Recipes and the 14-Day Carb Control Diet chapters.

End Your Day Right

As we have already established, it is very important to eat the right foods at the end of the day. Remember, you are not allowed to eat starches after 5 p.m. Instead you will be eating protein, fruit and vegetables, low-fat dairy products and essential fats in your evening meal. At the end of the book there are over 30 starch-free recipes for you to choose from – they will help you to put the Carb Curfew into practice and show you how easy it can be with a bit of know-how to keep your calorie intake in check.

The Carb Curfew 14-day Diet Plan chapter will also give you ideas for your evening meal.

Avoiding the Starches

What happens when the people you are with are eating starch and you can't because you are operating the Carb Curfew? Have a look at page 62 to see how you can make sensible food choices when you are faced with a situation where there is starch on the menu. The Carb Curfew gives you the flexibility to see what other foods you can eat and enjoy aside from starch, so you can continue to enjoy all your social activities and you are not put in the position where everyone can see that you are on a diet.

Chapter seven contains further advice about how to make good food choices when eating out in a variety of restaurants. Just because you are operating the Carb Curfew, it does not mean you cannot enjoy your evening meal. In fact, you will probably be surprised at just how many delicious starch-free dishes you can choose from the menu.

The Starch-Free Zone

There will be times when the Carb Curfew is out of the question – perhaps, for example, you are going to a dinner party at a friend's house and you know it's going to be virtually impossible to go starch-free. On these occasions, you can bring in the starch-free zone.

The starch-free zone means you say no to starch in your midday meal, thus freeing up your starch intake to have in your evening meal. If from time to time your lifestyle doesn't fit in with the Carb Curfew diet, don't beat yourself up about it – the Carb Curfew diet allows you to balance things out over time. We will talk more about this in chapter six and you will see how you can put the starch-free zone into practice in a variety of different scenarios.

Avoiding the Starches

Eating in a restaurant

Action points: say no to the bread basket; select a starch-free choice from the menu; request your dish to be served without potatoes, rice etc.

Suggested meal choice: smoked salmon (no bread) as a starter, grilled meat or fish with salad or vegetables as a main course and if you can't avoid dessert opt for fresh fruit sorbet

Eating at home by yourself or with partner

Action points: prepare evening meal with protein foods, pulses, vegetables and fruit

Suggested meal choice: Lime Marinated Grilled Salmon with Salsa (see page 201)

Eating at home with family

Action points: prepare starch-free main meal; cook starch (potatoes, rice or pasta) for rest of family

Suggested meal choice: Provencal-style Poached Chicken with Vegetables (see page 188). Serve with new potatoes and bread for the family

Entertaining guests

Action points: prepare a selection of dishes that are starch-free, but serve with speciality breads, rice and pastas as an additional extra. Make the vegetables and protein the main emphasis of the dish

Suggested meal choice: Chicken and Apricot Tagine (see page 183), served with green salad; or Prawn, Scallop and Parma Ham Kebabs with parsley salad (see page 203)

Success Story

Carolyn

Carolyn is a business woman who works long hours as well as leading a really hectic social life. Originally from Australia, she is determined to 'live it up' in London while she is working in England. Here is her story:

'Within eight months of arriving in London, I was experiencing substantial weight gain – this is something many foreigners suffer from having led physically active lives before arriving in the city and then sedentary lives once here. It concerned me so I attempted to lose this weight, but slowly I became extremely frustrated as I was making no progress. So I started the Carb Curfew plan and I can honestly say I felt the difference immediately. The biggest success factor for me was the Carb Curfew. It really helped me to stabilize my calorie intake – and at the same time it still allowed me to enjoy London and it didn't interfere with my social life.

Even within four weeks I had lost eight inches off my body and I continued to lose weight. The best part is that it is not only achievable but also fun. With such positive results it gives me the encouragement to keep going. The strategies have given me a new lease of life and I feel confident that I will be able to maintain it in the future.'

So how did Carolyn do?

Carolyn lost fourteen pounds in body weight – this meant she had dropped two dress sizes in just nine weeks.

Carolyn's Carb Curfew Menu Makeover

Breakfast
Before: 2 slices of toast with marmalade and butter, small glass orange juice, cup of tea
Now: 2 slices wholemeal toast with cottage cheese and glass orange juice or breakfast smoothie (see page 235)

Lunch
Before: jacket potato with baked beans
Now: small jacket potato with tuna and side salad

Snack
Before: a banana, thick slice of bread with fruit purée jam
Now: an apple

Dinner
Before: pasta with tomato sauce, grated cheese and garlic bread on the side, yoghurt for dessert

Now: 150g uncooked weight of lean meat or fish, served with green salad, broccoli and carrots, yoghurt with sliced fruit for dessert

A Final Word

So as we can see, the Carb Curfew is a great concept that allows you to eat the same food as your family, keep your calorie intake down, while boosting your intake of filling and healthy vegetables, pulses and fruit. You will find you have more energy throughout the day and you will wake up feeling less sluggish. So start applying the Carb Curfew now and you will soon feel the benefits whilst enjoying all your daily social activities. Don't worry if this seems a challenge at first – the recipes at the end of the book will help give you ideas and you will soon find you can adapt your meals quickly and easily, accommodating the whole family at the same time. Go on, start putting the Carb Curfew into practice today.

Take Action

- Start operating the Carb Curfew – begin this week.
- Draw up menu plans either from the suggested eating plans or the recipes at the end of the book.

◎ Plan ahead to see when you might need to implement a starch-free zone at lunchtime.

chapter four

Why More Water Means Less Fat

No natural resource is undervalued as much as water. These days most people do not drink nearly enough water. In fact, very many people never drink any at all and imagine that tea, coffee and fizzy drinks do much the same job, which they do not. It is very important to drink water to hydrate our bodies and flush out toxins and accumulated wastes from the system. If you drink less than eight glasses of water a day your body may be chronically dehydrated, you will lack energy and your brain can misinterpret this tiredness as a need to eat more food.

Feeling devoid of energy is one of the biggest challenges we face, especially when we are on a diet. So often we put a lack of energy down to not having eaten enough or slept enough, so we reach for a sugar fix for that instant energy boost. In fact, water has a greater impact on our energy levels than any other nutrient. So when we are tired we need to address how well-hydrated our body is first to ensure we are providing the right environment for all our body's own metabolic responses to work effectively.

Why is Water Important?

Water plays a vital role in enabling our body to function properly. It is especially important for weight management because it swells food cells and helps our body absorb vital nutrients. Water makes us feel more satisfied with the food we have eaten because it bulks it up, thus stretching the stomach wall and sending messages to the brain telling us we are full. Also, the water content in blood helps the absorption and transportation of all the nutrients, vitamins and minerals in the body and helps flush out all the waste products from the system. When you change to a healthier diet your body will initially pro-duce more toxins and you will need to rid the body of these with water.

So a vital part of the Carb Curfew diet plan is to drink more water. In this chapter you'll learn about the effect of different drinks on your body and how to:

- Get out of the habit of drinking too many of the wrong sort of drinks.
- Get into the habit of giving your body the water it needs.

Carb Curfew Essentials

The three keys to successful hydration are:

1. Drink a minimum of two litres (eight glasses) of water a day, spread evenly throughout the day.
2. No more than two cups of coffee or tea or two cans of fizzy drink a day.
3. No more than ten units of alcohol a week.

Are You Drinking Enough Water?

To help you find out what your hydration levels are like, answer the following questions.

1. What colour is your urine?
   a. dark yellow
   b. yellow
   c. almost clear

2. When did you last have a drink of water?
   a. more than two hours ago
   b. one to two hours ago
   c. within the last hour

3. How often do you go to the toilet in the day?
   a. less than twice
   b. two to four times
   c. more than four times

4. How many cups of tea/coffee/fizzy drinks do you drink a day?
   a. five plus
   b. two to five
   c. one to two

5. How many glasses of water do you drink a day?
   a. one to four
   b. four to eight
   c. eight to twelve

6. How often do you feel thirsty?
   a. never
   b. sometimes
   c. frequently

7. When you drink alcohol do you drink water as well?
   a. never
   b. sometimes
   c. always

If you answered:

Mostly A
If you scored mostly A you are probably unaware of the importance of water. It is likely that you are acutely dehydrated, which means you lack the appropriate amount of water for your body to function properly both when exercising and in everyday life. This is putting a lot of pressure on your system, which in turn will have a direct impact on your energy levels without you even realizing it.

Take action now. Cut down your tea and coffee intake to a maximum of two cups a day. Drink a glass of water immediately after exercise and sip water during exercise sessions. Start to build up your water intake to two litres a day. Begin by adding two glasses of water to your existing intake and add an extra glass each week until you reach your quota.

Mostly B
If you scored mostly B you are aware of the importance of water but you still have a little way to go to bring your body up to its right hydration state. It is likely that

your body is in a state where it is never fully hydrated to meet the demands placed on it day in and day out. The water you are drinking should be better spread out during the day to help hydrate your body consistently.

You need to focus on increasing your water intake to eight glasses a day. Spread these out throughout the day to avoid excess stress on your bladder and the need to rush to the toilet the whole time.

Mostly C

If you scored mostly C you are doing a good job of fulfilling your hydration needs. Your body is starting to tell you when you need to drink and replenish your fluids. Work on increasing your intake of fluids at the start of the day. This will have an immediate effect on your energy levels to set you up for the day. Plan to hit your water intake of eight glasses each day, whatever the circumstances and spread the water intake evenly throughout the day.

How to Check Your Hydration Status

1. Look! Your urine should be a very pale yellow straw colour.
2. Taking vitamin supplements will affect the colour of your urine. To get a true colour reading, pass water twice after taking the supplements before checking the colour of your urine.

3. Check your body weight. Weigh yourself before
    your usual exercise session and establish a baseline
    weight before exercise. Weigh yourself immedi-
    ately after your exercise session – every pound
    lost in weight equals a loss of two cups of fluid.
    You will then need to replace this loss of fluid by
    drinking water. Do not fall into the trap of thinking
    this decrease in weight is a loss of body fat.
    Unfortunately body fat takes longer than a one-
    hour exercise session to disappear!

The Low-Down on Hydration
How Much Water Should I Drink?

It is generally agreed that we all need two litres of water
a day. This figure is the minimum – if you exercise a lot,
travel, have a high fibre diet, live in a hot climate or work
in an air-conditioned office your water intake should be
higher, at least two and a half litres a day. And if you think
that's a lot consider the advice professional athletes are
given – in hot weather it's eight litres a day.

You can drink either tap water or mineral water,
whichever you prefer – drinking too much sparkling mineral water however might cause stomach discomfort.

Can I Drink All My Water in One Go?

It is much better to space out the fluid you drink throughout the day. Imagine your body as a plant in a flowerpot which has not been watered properly for a few weeks. Its leaves are drooping and it is looking rather sorry for itself. The plant clearly needs water but if we watered it with all of the water it needs in one go, then the water would flow out the bottom of the flowerpot and very little would be retained by the soil to feed the plant. However, if the same amount of water is fed to the plant little by little, allowing the plant to absorb the water, then the plant will hydrate back to its former glory. The same concept applies with the body. If we go too long without consuming the proper amount of fluid and then we consume it all in one go, the bladder and kidneys have to work exceptionally hard and we will just end up making frequent visits to the toilet as most of the water will pass straight through us, rather than being retained as needed in the body.

Why Do I Rarely Feel Thirsty?

If you rarely feel thirsty it is likely that the message centre in your brain that tells you when you are thirsty has become lazy and has lost the ability to give you the right message that you need to drink. Quite simply, your body has got so used to being chronically dehydrated that this is now its normal state. In addition, the hydration message centre is very close to the hunger message centre in the brain, so it is likely that any messages you are receiving will be interpreted as you needing to eat rather than needing to drink. The good news is that you can re-educate or retrain your brain so your thirst mechanism centre starts to tell you to drink again. By gradually increasing your water intake you will find that over a period of as little as three weeks your body will start to tell you when you need to drink water.

When you next feel like eating something, ask yourself the question: Am I hungry or am I thirsty? Always drink a glass of water before you start to eat something. As I said at the start of the chapter, water is especially important for weight management as it swells food cells and helps our body absorb vital nutrients.

Did You Know?

New research shows that drinking a cup of black, unsweetened coffee or green tea just before aerobic exercise can actually improve your workout as the caffeine will boost your body's energy release mechanisms.

Do Tea or Coffee Count Towards My Daily Water Intake?

You may think that cups of tea and coffee boost your daily water intake. Unfortunately this is not the case as they are diuretics and actually encourage your body to get rid of fluid. Even though they are a liquid and do contain water they dehydrate the body rather than effectively providing the cells with the fluid they need.

Does This Mean I Can Never Drink Tea and Coffee?

No. For many people tea and coffee are an integral part of the day and there is really no need to forgo them completely. But your intake does need to be moderated. The Carb Curfew diet plan recommends no more than two cups of tea or coffee a day. These two cups do not go towards your quota of two litres of water a day, so you need to make sure you fulfil your water quota as well.

Studies have shown that drinking tea and coffee can have a mild health benefit. For example, a single cup of tea, with or without milk, provides a useful source of flavonoids, which act as antioxidants and can help to protect the body against heart disease and cancer. Green tea, which is very popular in Asia, has the highest concentration of flavonoids. But remember, even though there are health benefits, tea and coffee contain tannin and caffeine, which can inhibit the absorption of the essential nutrients calcium and iron. You should also be aware that if you have a cup of tea or coffee in the morning with a multivitamin tablet, the tannins and caffeine can inhibit the absorption of essential nutrients.

But It's So Bland!

If the taste of water doesn't do anything for you, then you can flavour the water with a twist of lime or lemon or add a splash of freshly squeezed orange juice. Alternatively, you can add a slice of lemon and a chunk of fresh ginger to hot water (this is particularly cleansing first thing in the morning).

Fruit juice cordials can be a great way to make your water intake a little more interesting – but do watch the calorie content. For example, a 250ml glass of pink grapefruit squash made with one part juice and 4 parts water will give 88 calories. Hit your 2 litre quota of 8 glasses of this, and that is a whopping 704 calories without you even eating anything! Reduced sugar and low-calorie cordials can help you keep the calories down while helping to boost your fluid intake but always have a look at the labels for hidden calories that can sneak up on you without you realizing. In addition, some of these cordial drinks can contain a lot of artificial sweeteners, which are not necessarily as healthy for you as natural sugars. So the general rule is, if you need to flavour your water with cordials keep them weak to act as a hint of taste rather than a concentrated flavour burst. Diluted cordials are especially helpful when you need to hydrate your body after exercise.

Herbal teas can be another great way to boost your fluid intake, though not all are stimulant-free. Some herbal teas such as fennel and dandelion are particularly good to drink because they contain properties that can assist in ridding your body of toxins. So drinking herbal teas can contribute towards your two-litre target. However, because water really is the gold standard, a good tip to follow is to make five of your eight glasses of fluid a day WATER.

Is it Okay to Drink Alcohol?

For many of us alcohol is a pleasurable part of our lives. But whether we like it or not, alcohol is a major hindrance to long-term fat loss and weight management. This is for two reasons:

1. Alcohol provides a lot of empty calories that have no nutritional value for the body. It provides seven calories per gram, which will significantly increase your total calorie intake if you consume large quantities. In addition, many alcoholic drinks contain sugars and other carbohydrates which increase your calorie intake further.

2. Calories from alcohol, unlike the energy we derive from carbohydrate, protein and fat, cannot be stored by the body. This means that any calories we consume from alcohol have to be burnt off by the body before the body can burn off calories from other sources of food – no matter how nutritious these foods might be. Any excess calories that haven't been burnt off during the day, regardless of where they have come from, will simply be stored as fat in the fat cells. Remember, the fat cells have the capacity to keep on getting bigger and bigger!

Watch Out For Those Wines!

Jane was suffering from middle-age spread. She had always dieted and generally watched her weight, however as she got older she became extra determined to keep her body fat levels under control. She religiously watched her fat intake and operated a Carb Curfew but she was overlooking one thing – the amount of wine she was drinking. The two glasses she drank at the end of her day while she unwound before her evening meal soon became a total of five by the end of the evening. By the end of the week this meant Jane was easily consuming an extra 500 calories a day without her really noticing it. Jane says:

'As soon as I understood how all these calories were adding up from alcohol and how my body was not able to use them, I was able to see where I had been going astray. I have now cut back and I drink more spritzers which help me hydrate at the same time. I have also found that I snack a lot less as I have more willpower to avoid nibbles like cashew nuts and crisps.'

So how did Jane do?
Over the course of ten weeks Jane dropped eight pounds of body fat and she fitted into her favourite skirt, which had been left unworn at the back of her wardrobe for over four years. The extra vitality she felt in the mornings also helped Jane to be more active throughout the day.

So How Much Alcohol Can I Drink?

Doctors recommend that safe drinking levels are between 21 and 28 units per week for men and between 14 and 21 units for women. One unit is a glass of wine, a single measure of spirit or half a pint of normal strength beer.

Some research has shown that moderate drinking – one to two units a day – can actually do you some good as it helps to counteract cardiovascular disease. This works by preventing the blood from clotting, a risk factor leading to heart disease and strokes. However, these benefits only apply to people who are already at risk of heart disease. For women who have not gone through the menopause and men under 40, heavy drinking (more than 10 units at a time) is linked with significantly raised blood pressure.

Because of the calories contained in alcohol the Carb Curfew diet plan recommends no more than 10 units of alcohol a week. These should be spread out over the course of the week rather than being consumed all in one evening. This would put extra pressure on your kidneys and, more importantly, create a large increase in your daily average intake of calories. Being consistent with your daily calorie and fat gram intake is a crucial factor in your long-term success (see chapter six for more about this).

Some alcoholic drinks contain more calories than others: a single measure of brandy, whisky, gin, rum or vodka contains 50 calories; champagne contains 70 calories per unit; white wine and red wine contain 75 and 90 calories per unit respectively; bottled beer contains 90 calories per unit, and alcopops are the worst offenders with a whopping 215 calories per one to two units.

Alcohol also has a significant dehydrating effect – far more marked than tea and coffee. If you drink alcohol you must ensure you top up your daily water consumption to balance out its effect. If you drink alcohol after exercise in hot weather you will notice the effect of dehydration even more. You'll take frequent visits to the bathroom and lose valuable fluids. More importantly, it will trigger off your thirst mechanism which may act as a stimulus for you to eat more when really it is water you need to be consuming.

Juices and Smoothies

Fruit juices and smoothies can be a quick and easy way to boost your energy levels and hydrate your body. They are also a great way to help you get your five portions of fruit and vegetables a day.

Fruit juices are high in antioxidants, which help to prevent disease and premature ageing. You need to drink fruit juices within two hours of making them for them to be of the most nutritional value. A glass of freshly squeezed orange juice may be as far as you get or you may really get the juicing bug and invest in a juice extractor. Here are some tasty fruit combinations to try – remember to always dilute your juices with a little water to boost your water intake and aid your body's ability to absorb the nutrients:

- asparagus, carrot and cucumber
- kiwi, mango and orange juice
- apple and grape
- apple, carrot, melon and ginger
- tomato, red pepper and cucumber
- carrot, tomato and beetroot
- apple, orange and strawberry

- apple, pineapple and papaya
- apple, asparagus and watercress

Fruit smoothies are also great thirst quenchers and they provide an excellent breakfast on the go or a fantastic energy boost in the middle of the afternoon. Some commercial smoothies can be high in calories as full-fat yoghurt and milks are often added – so always have a quick look at the label before buying one or ask how they are made if you are in a juice bar.

To add some creaminess to your smoothies without piling on additional calories, pour your favourite low-fat fruit yoghurts into an ice-cube tray and freeze. You can then take out the cubes and add them to your smoothie. Alternatively, for speed, you could freeze the whole yoghurt and peel off the container when you are ready to use.

The following recipe is a great start to your day:

Creamy Berry Smoothie

handful of frozen fruit (I find the bags of frozen fruits of the forest from the frozen fruit section of the supermarket particularly good)

1/2 pint skimmed milk or soya milk

1/2 tablespoon wheatgerm

4 cubes frozen fruits of the forest low-fat yoghurt

ice cubes

Put all your ingredients in a blender and liquidize for about 30 seconds. Pour into a glass and drink. Add a little water if you find the consistency too thick. For a change, try frozen peach yoghurt cubes.

Note: You can use either skimmed milk or soya milk in your smoothies. Both skimmed milk and unsweetened organic soya milk provide similar calorie values of 34 and 36 calories per 100ml respectively. Soya milk, as well as being lactose and cholesterol-free, is rich in plant phyto-oestrogens, which have been shown to have a protective effect against some reproductive cancers. So while soya milk may not be everyone's favourite it does have huge health benefits – consuming it in the form of a smoothie where its taste is disguised can be a convenient way to boost your daily phyto-oestrogen intake. If you really can't stand the idea of soya milk try these other good phyto-oestrogen sources: yam, black-eyed peas, liquorice root drunk as tea, kale and dandelion greens.

See the 14-Day Carb Control Diet chapter for more about smoothies.

Carb Curfew Hydration Makeover

Before Sarah started the Carb Curfew plan she was struggling with her weight and lacking in energy. She worked in a busy office where the tea trolley and cafeteria were always on hand. The Carb Curfew plan alerted her to the fact that she needed to address her hydration levels. She started recording her fluid intake over a week, noting what she was drinking, how much and when. She could quickly see she was consuming far too much tea and coffee, which she partly did to keep her hunger at bay. At first Sarah thought she would never be able to drink two litres of water a day but with a little bit of effort she was hitting her quota after three weeks.

Sarah's Strategy

Instead of her usual cup of tea on waking Sarah had a cup of hot water with a slice of lemon. She continued to have a cup of coffee or tea with her breakfast but also had a glass of water. Sarah's mid-morning cup of tea was replaced with a cup of herbal tea and instead of drinking a can of diet soda with her lunch she had two glasses of water. Her mid-afternoon cuppa was replaced with some diluted fruit juice and instead of her usual 2 glasses of wine and cappuccino at dinner she had one glass of wine and two glasses of water. All this meant that Sarah's caffeine intake dropped from 350g per day to 50g and her total fluid intake was transformed from two units of alcohol and no water whatsoever to one unit of alcohol and two litres of water.

And the result – Sarah felt a marked improvement in her energy levels, she felt better able to concentrate at work and her appetite decreased.

Carb Curfew Hydration Tips

◎ Invest in a pull-top drink canister. Fill this up with water and keep it topped up in the car. Drinking water while sitting in traffic is a great way to keep your fluid levels topped up.

◎ When you are in the kitchen have a glass of water on your work surface and drink it as you prepare a meal.

◎ Aim to drink a glass of water first thing in the morning then consume three-quarters of a litre by lunchtime. Spreading your water consumption over the day avoids putting too much pressure on the bladder.

Changing Your Drinking Habits

Throughout the day there are ways you can change your drinking habits to make sure you drink the right amount of water. Here are some suggestions – use those that are most appropriate to your daily routine:

◎ start your day with a cup of hot water with a slice of lemon

◎ drink 2 glasses of water with your breakfast

o
the)
up the

⊚ replace m
  green tea

⊚ always have a

⊚ start serving and

⊚ drink a glass of wat
  drink

⊚ drink a glass of water m   nd-
  afternoon

⊚ measure out 2 litres of water   the start of the day
  and aim to have drunk all of it by 9 p.m.

⊚ always pour yourself a glass of water when drinking
  your daily 2 cups of tea or coffee

⊚ get out of the habit of drinking tea/coffee every time
  you complete a task. Replace with herbal tea or
  water

⊚ start your day with a fruit smoothie to help boost
  energy and hydration levels straight away

⊚ buy a bottle of water on your way to work every
  morning. Have it on your desk and drink throughout
  the day

...d drunk a lot
...ter before going to

...ter before you eat anything
...habit of asking yourself every time you
...something to eat: Am I hungry or am I really
thirsty?
◎ experiment with fruit smoothies to boost energy
levels mid-afternoon and help you hydrate

Tips from Successful Carb Cutters

Catherine
'I have two glass jars on my sideboard, one empty and one with eight small pebbles. My aim is to fill the empty jar with the pebbles. Every time I have a glass of water I transfer one of the pebbles from the full jar to the empty jar. It works as a great motivator for me and helps me keep track of exactly how many glasses of water I have actually drunk.'

Alexandra
'Drinking loads of water really does stop you feeling the need to binge. What I found very helpful was the suggestion of going out of the kitchen and doing something else if that binge feeling reared its ugly head and/or keeping a jug of water in the fridge plus a whole load of peeled carrots and rice cakes to nibble in emergencies.'

A Final Word

So now you have read about the benefits of drinking enough water and seen how you can make small simple changes to your daily routine to make sure your body stays properly hydrated. This is probably the easiest part of the Carb Curfew diet plan – but it is a key strategy. Stick to the following action points and you'll be well on the way to a super-hydrated and less hungry body.

Take Action

- Start every day with a cup of hot water and lemon.
- Commit yourself to increasing your water intake. Aim to have a glass of water on waking, one glass at breakfast, two glasses mid-morning, one at lunch, two mid-afternoon, and a glass with your evening meal.
- When you feel hungry, get into the habit of asking yourself: 'Am I hungry or am I really thirsty?'
- Always drink a glass of water before eating something.

chapter five

Fats –
The Good and the Bad

Ask any seasoned dieter what they need to do to lose weight and they'll tell you, 'cut out the fat'. We are right to be aware of the role fat has in helping us address our weight and body fat goals, but focusing solely on the amount of fat we consume does not provide us with the complete picture. It is the total amount of calories we consume in conjunction with the amount of fat and the type of fat that is vital to our success.

The fat in our food is the most concentrated source of energy. One gram of fat provides us with over twice as many calories as one gram of either protein or carbohydrate. Studies show that if we want to lose weight both our calorie intake and the number of calories we consume from fat are important. However, it is important to stress that some fat is important for good health. Certain foods which contain fat supply the fat-soluble vitamins A, D, E and K and some essential fats that our bodies cannot make for themselves. If we cut out all the fat in our diet we would be depriving our bodies of some very important nutrients.

So the next strategy is to figure out fats. In this chapter you'll learn about the role of fat and its impact on the body and how to:

◎ Cut down on your overall saturated fat intake
◎ Increase the essential functional fats in your diet
◎ Learn how to read food labels

Carb Curfew Essentials

The two key rules to make fat work for you are:

1. Reduce your overall fat intake to around 40 grams a day.
2. Make sure you have at least 15 grams of the right fats in your diet a day.

Do You Know Your Fats?

Answer the following questions to help you find out how much fat and which types of fat you are currently eating.

1. Do you always buy reduced-fat products?
   a. yes
   b. no
2. Do you consume three servings of oily fish a week?
   a. yes
   b. no
3. Which of the following cooking methods do you mostly use?
   a. steam, grill, poach
   b. stir-fry, fry, deep-fry
4. Do you eat cheese on most days?
   a. no
   b. yes
5. Do you use olive oil liberally believing it to be healthy?
   a. yes
   b. no
6. Do you try to cut all fat out of your diet thinking it is the best way to lose weight?
   a. no
   b. yes

If you answered:

Mostly A

You are aware of the fat content of foods; however it is likely that you are not getting enough of the right essential fats. In addition, you may perceive that your overall fat intake is low but the quantity of the lower fat versions you are consuming may be large. Alternatively, you may be adding additional calories to your daily intake by consuming excess olive oil. As you will see later in the chapter, even though olive oil is a healthy fat it still provides 47 calories per teaspoon. Read your food labels and be aware of the amount of olive oil and other oils you are consuming in dressings and stir-frying.

Mostly B

Your total fat intake is likely to be high due to your intake of visible fats and invisible fats. In addition, it is likely you are consuming a greater proportion of saturated fat, which is associated with an increased risk of heart disease and clogging of the arteries (atherosclerosis). Cut down your overall intake of fat by reducing the amount of visible fats you are consuming. In addition, aim to consume three servings of oily fish a week.

Visible and Invisible Fats

As we discussed in chapter two, visible fats are foods that contain an obvious fat content. The fat we see on meat, as well as foods such as butter, lard, cream and oils are all examples of visible fats.

Invisible fats are foods that do not have an apparent fat content. These fats may make up some of the ingredients in a recipe or they may be found in specific foods with a naturally high fat content that we are often unaware of. Chocolate, avocado, coconut and taramasalata are all examples of foods containing invisible fats.

The Different Types of Fat

All fats provide nine calories per gram, but the different fats perform certain functions in the body and consequently the health qualities of each fat are quite different.

Saturated Fats

Saturated fats are non-essential fats. As I mentioned earlier, eating too much saturated fat is associated with an increased risk of heart disease and atherosclerosis. These fats do not play a healthy role in the body – in fact, when we consume a diet high in saturated fat the simplest thing for our body to do with it is to transport it to the fat cells and dump it there. Quite simply, the fat cells welcome the saturated fat we eat with open arms and our fat cells get bigger and bigger, our shape gets larger and larger, our clothes get tighter and tighter and our health risks get higher and higher. Butter, lard, cheese and fat on meat are all examples of saturated fat.

Trans Fats

Trans fats are also non-essential fats as they have no functional health role to play in the body. They are man-made fats produced during hydrogenation of vegetable oil – a process used in the manufacture of various foodstuffs such as margarine. Their consumption is associated with an increased risk of both cancer and heart disease. The majority of trans fats in the diet come from processed foods – look for the word hydrogenated on your food labels and you have found trans fats.

Polyunsaturated Fats

Polyunsaturated fats have a very important health role to play in the body, such as helping to decrease blood cholesterol levels. Polyunsaturated fats are divided into two groups – omega-3 essential fatty acids and omega-6 essential fatty acids. They are considered to be 'essential' because we are unable to manufacture them in the body.

Omega-3 essential fatty acids are found mainly in fish oils as well as flax seeds and pumpkin seeds. Salmon, herring, sardines, trout, pilchards and mackerel are all good sources of omega-3 fats – tuna fish is not such a good source of omega-3 but as a low-fat alternative to meat and cheese it is a healthy option for the family. It is widely believed that omega-3 essential fats help prevent atherosclerosis and help lower blood pressure and triglyceride levels. Omega-3 fats make blood platelets less sticky and less likely to clog, thus decreasing the risk of artery blockage and heart attack. Eating three servings of oily fish a week or using flax seed oil as part of your salad dressing will help you hit your omega-3 fatty acid quota.

Omega-6 essential fatty acids are found mainly in hemp, pumpkin, sunflower, safflower, sesame and corn oil. About half of the oils found in these seeds are from omega-6 fatty acids. Omega-6 fatty acids, like omega-3 fatty acids, have an important function in the body. They are involved in preventing blood clots, lowering blood pressure, helping to maintain the water balance in the body and helping the body to stabilize blood sugar levels.

So as you can see, both of these fats are very important for our bodies. In addition, they actually help us burn protein, carbohydrate and fat. This means that if the fats we eat are from these essential fat sources they will play an important role in the healthy functioning of our bodies before what is left of them is transported to the fat cells and stored.

Cooking With Fats

Be careful when cooking with polyunsaturated fats – they can become damaged when heated at high temperatures, which decreases their health benefits. Monounsaturated fats such as olive oil are a better choice to cook with because they are more stable than polyunsaturated fats.

Monounsaturated Fats

Monounsaturated fats have been coined the most healthy fats, partly because research has shown that the 'Mediterranean diet', with its high olive oil content, can help lower cholesterol levels and prevent heart disease. However, what we fail to remember is that a tablespoon of olive oil will give us the same amount of calories as a tablespoon of melted lard! So the total amount of fat is still important. Sources of monounsaturated fat include olive oil and rapeseed oil.

So we have established so far, you do need to cut down on your overall fat intake, especially your saturated fats, but we have also seen that some fats are good fats and are in fact very important for our health.

All About Fats

Saturated Fats (non-essential)

Typical sources: meat, dairy products and some tropical oils including palm oil and cocoa butter

How do I spot them?: generally solid at room temperature, e.g. butter, cheese, coconut oil

Health effects: increases cholesterol levels; increases risk of heart disease and certain cancers

Advice: the less the better – should make up no more than 8 per cent of total calories

Trans Fats (non-essential)

Typical sources: margarine, shortening, fried foods, breads, crackers, snack foods, spreads, processed/ready-prepared foods

How do I spot them?: look for the term hydrogenated or partially-hydrogenated fat on food labels – often found in low-fat spreads

Health effects: has a negative effect on cholesterol levels; may increase risk of heart disease and breast cancer

Advice: the less the better, minimize consumption. Avoid products that use the words 'hydrogenated' or 'partially hydrogenated' on the food label

Monounsaturated (essential)

Typical sources: olive (preferably cold pressed), rape-seed, canola, almond, cashew, hazelnut, macadamia, pecan and peanut oils

How do I spot them?: generally liquid at room temperature

Health effects: beneficial effect on cholesterol levels; lowers bad blood fats and increases good blood fats; helps prevent heart disease

Advice: olive oil and rapeseed oil are your best choices. These should make up 12 per cent of total calories

Polyunsaturated Fats (made up of omega-6 and omega-3 essential fatty acids)

Typical sources: vegetable oils and fish and fish oils

How do I spot them?: generally liquid at room temperature

Health effects: helps prevent atherosclerosis (furring of the arteries); helps lower blood pressure and cholesterol levels

Advice: these are the healthier fats, but should make up no more than 10 per cent of total calories

Omega-6 Essential Fatty Acids

Typical sources: corn, safflower, sesame, soybean and sunflower oils, nuts and wheatgerm

How do I spot them?: the extracted oils of these foods are liquid

Health effects: thought to boost the immune system, but watch out as too much vegetable oil can alter the delicate balance of omega-6 and omega-3 fats

Advice: limit consumption of these vegetable oils. Mayonnaise and salad dressings are often made with these – substitute with olive, canola and flax seed oil

Omega-3 Essential Fatty Acids

Typical sources: cold water fish (salmon, mackerel, herring, halibut, tuna and sardines), flax seed, hemp seed, walnuts and their oils, canola and soybean oils, green leafy vegetables

How do I spot them?: the visible strands of fat on these fish are rich in omega-3 fats

Health effects: inhibits blood clots; reduces risk of heart disease; increases immune function

Advice: most people will need to increase consumption to reach the ideal 3.6g daily

---

Watch the Oil!

One teaspoon of oil provides 5 grams of fat and 47 calories. One tablespoon of oil provides 15 grams of fat and 141 calories.

The Low-Down on Fat

Why Do We Need to Eat Fat?

Although most of us eat far too much fat in our daily diet, we do need some. Here are some reasons why:

- All types of fat give us nine calories per gram so it provides a valuable source of energy.
- It helps the body produce key hormones that regulate various bodily processes.
- It helps transport and absorb carotenoids, a group of powerful antioxidants, and the fat-soluble vitamins A, D, E and K.
- It gives us our shape and a glow of health as opposed to looking gaunt and bony.
- It acts as a thermal blanket, keeping us warm and defending the body against heat loss.

How Much Fat Should We Eat a Day?

It is often recommended that fat intake should be no more than 30 per cent of the total calories eaten each day. But percentages can be misleading – 3 per cent of a 5,000 calorie diet is a lot more than 30 per cent of a 1,500 calorie diet. Although percentages can give us a useful rough guideline, the most important thing is to keep track of the total amount of fat grams you are eating in your diet. The Carb Curfew diet plan recommends a daily fat intake of

40 grams and a calorie intake range of between 1,200-1,500, dependent upon your activity levels, diet history and stage on the plan.

The Carb Curfew diet plan will help you keep track of your fat gram intake. The recipe section is full of foods and meal ideas that will help you stay within your 40-gram fat budget. You can also learn a lot about your total fat intake by reading food labels to check the amount of fat in the product. Some labels will even specify the types of fats.

Will I Still Lose Weight if I Cut Down on Calories But Not Fat?

While you may initially lose weight, if you cut down on your calories but you still have a high fat intake you will experience frustration at not reaching the weight you want to be. This is because you will still have more fat in your diet than your body is able to use and the easiest thing for the body to do is to store it as body fat in the ever-adaptable fat cells. In addition, it is likely that you will feel hungry as the volume of food you consume will actually be quite small due to the fact that fat has such a high calorie value for the amount consumed.

If I Eat Only Reduced Fat or Low-fat Products Will I Lose Weight?

While the aim is to keep the total amount of fat down and purchasing reduced fat versions of regular food may seem a convenient way to achieve this, studies have shown that individuals who think they are eating low-fat products actually consume more of them because they think they can thus push up their total calorie intake. So spreading your bread with an extra thick layer of low-fat cream cheese is no different from spreading the same piece of bread with a thin layer of regular fat cream cheese. So if you hate the idea of eating reduced fat versions of regular foods then your strategy should be to eat the normal product but watch the amount you eat.

Hidden Fat Grams in Everyday Snacks

You might be surprised at just how much fat is contained in the fast foods we love to snack on. Some of the snacks listed below will actually use up half a whole day's Carb Curfew fat budget in one go.

Snacks and Grams of Fat Per Portion

packet of crisps (30g bag)	9
slice of hot-buttered toast – butter oozing off!	10
2 cream crackers with a wedge of Cheddar cheese	20
slice of pepperoni pizza	10

1 pitta bread with a serving of taramasalata	30
bar of chocolate (50g bar)	15
packet of peanuts (50g packet)	25
1 scone	7
1 bagel	2
1 rice cake	0.5
piece of fruit	trace

Remember, fat grams are not the whole story – total calories are also important (the Carb Curfew will help you here). But the selection of what you nibble on can really affect your daily fat gram budget. But don't despair. For all those fat-filled foods we love to eat, there are plenty of healthier, lower fat alternatives available. Going low-fat certainly doesn't have to mean sacrificing flavour either. Have a look at this range of high-fat foods and their healthier lower fat substitutes.

Low-Fat Alternatives to High-Fat Foods

Foods and Grams of Fat Per Portion

cream

double cream (1 tablespoon)	14
double cream, half-fat (1 tablespoon)	7
single cream (1 tablespoon)	8
natural bio yoghurt (150g pot)	4
yoghurt – low-fat, plain (150g pot)	0.3
fromage frais – low-fat (1 tablespoon)	0.05
fat-free Greek yoghurt (1 tablespoon)	0

chips

thin cut (burger-bar portion – approx 125g)	22
thick cut (fish and chip shop portion – approx 250g)	35
oven (200g)	7
baked potato, large	0.1

pork chop

grilled with fat left on (165g)	21
grilled with fat removed (135g)	9

cod

fried in batter	9
poached	1

chicken (100g)

roast meat (light and dark), with skin	14
roast dark meat, no skin	7
roast breast meat, no skin	4

turkey (100g)

roast breast meat, with skin	6.5
roast breast meat, no skin	1.4
roast dark meat, no skin	4.1

cheese

Cheddar (50g)	17
Edam (50g)	12
low-fat Cheddar (50g)	8

cottage cheese (2 tablespoons)	1.5
mini cheese spread triangle	4

milk (one cup)
whole	8
semi-skimmed	3.2
skimmed	0.2

spreads (enough to cover one piece of bread but not too thick)
butter	8
margarine	8
low-fat spread	3
cream cheese	2.8
reduced fat cream cheese	1.6
quark	0.3

dips (1 heaped tablespoon)
taramasalata	23
hummus	11
guacamole	8
tzatziki	4
sour cream onion dip	7

mayo (1 heaped teaspoon)
mayo	12
reduced fat mayo	4.5

breads

croissant, medium	12
focaccia (75 g)	4
1 crumpet, medium	0.3
1 potato cake, medium	1
1 bagel, large	2
1 pitta	2
slice wholemeal bread	1
slice of ryvita	0.7

Carb Curfew Healthy Fats Makeover

Heather, a busy mum, turned to the Carb Curfew diet plan when her weight-loss efforts were not paying dividends. Heather was conscious about her weight but she was also careful not to give the wrong example to her children about weight loss by going on fad diets or being fussy with her food. Consequently, Heather's diet was fairly balanced but she did need to cut down on the amount of fat she was consuming. I encouraged Heather to write down what she ate for a week and quite soon we were able to identify several high-fat culprits that made a regular appearance. This is Heather's revamped healthy fats eating plan:

Breakfast
Before: 2 slices toast with butter and marmalade, cup of coffee
Now: Swiss muesli with live bio yoghurt

Lunch
Before: jacket potato with butter and sweetcorn, side salad with mayo
Now: open sardine green salad sandwich (no mayo)

Mid-afternoon snack
Before: 50g chocolate bar
Now: Creamy Berry Smoothie (see page 83)

Dinner
Before: lasagne with salad dressing and garlic bread, ice cream
Now: Provencal-style Poached Chicken with Vegetables (see page 188), fruit salad

Heather was really pleased with her makeover – not only did she have more energy but she felt really confident that she was giving her children a positive message about healthy eating while she achieved her body fat goals. She particularly enjoyed the smoothie, which she had while the children had their tea.

So how did Heather do?

Over twelve weeks Heather lost two inches off her waist and two inches off her belly button measurements and she decreased her body fat by three per cent, which brought her body fat into the healthy body fat range for her age.

In the Kitchen

It's not just the individual ingredients and the types of food we eat that make a difference. Different ways of preparing foods can also have a big impact on the final fat gram count of each meal.

Cooking Methods and Lower Fat Alternatives

Frying
Lower fat alternative: bake, steam, grill

Stir-frying
Lower fat alternative: blanch vegetables in boiling water first and then flash stir-fry in seasoning

Stews and casseroles
Lower fat alternative: brown off the meat first in a small amount of liquid, or prepare dish a day ahead of serving and skim off fat from top of the dish

Deep-fat frying

Lower fat alternative: experiment with microwaving and en papillote – a method of cooking in which food is wrapped in greaseproof paper or foil and baked in the oven. Works well with vegetables and seafood. Adding a little liquid such as citrus juices or wine and herbs can help keep food moist as well as adding flavour

Roasting

Lower fat alternative: can be a no-fat cooking method – use a metal stand (trivet) to help fat drain away from food. If basting is required, try brushing with oil to reduce the quantity used and mix with balsamic and sherry vinegar to make a small amount of oil go further

Carb Curfew Cooking Tips

- Purchase a good sharp knife to trim all visible fat from food prior to cooking.
- Pour olive oil or flax seed oil into a spray canister and use to spritz salads and lightly grease pans.
- Remove all visible fat from meat before cooking.
- Invest in a good-quality non-stick pan.
- Blanch veggies in boiling water prior to stir-frying – this minimizes the fat you will require in the stir-fry pan and the vegetables will retain more of their nutritional value while absorbing minimum fat.

Reading Food Labels

If you really want to get your fats sorted you will need to get into the habit of examining food labels. These days all packaged foods are required to carry detailed labels explaining the nutritional value of the product. A typical food label will look something like this:

Average Values	per 100g	per 300g serving
Energy	305kj	915kj
	70kcal	210kcal
Protein	6.1g	18.3g
Carbohydrate,	9.6g	28.8g
of which sugars	0.8g	2.4g
Fat,	1.9g	5.7g
of which saturates	0.6g	1.8g
Fibre	1.2g	3.6g
Sodium	0.25g	0.75g

The amount of energy in a product is shown as kcal and kj. Kcal or kilocalories are the same as calories; kj or kilo-joules are simply another way of measuring energy. Here is how you read a food label:

⊙ At the top of the label you will see the information is presented in per 100 grams and per serving. I always advise looking at the per serving information because you have to do less arithmetic and this is actually what you will be putting in your mouth.

◎ Look at the total amount of calories. In this example, the food will provide 210 calories per serving.

◎ Look at the total amount of fat per serving. This product will provide you with 5.7 grams per serving.

◎ Look at the amount of saturated fat. This product provides 1.8 grams of saturated fat.

◎ Next check out the list of ingredients. Avoid ingredients such as hydrogenated or partially hydrogenated vegetable oils and trans fats. As a rule of thumb, the higher up the ingredient list these fats appear the more of them there will be in the product.

Verdict

Total calorie content is 210, total fat intake is 5.7 grams of which 1.8 grams are saturated. Remember your total daily fat budget is around 40 grams so this product is a good selection. It is actually an example of a ready-prepared meal – serve it with three portions of vegetables and a dessert of fresh fruit and natural bio yoghurt and you have yourself a very balanced meal that fulfils your fat gram criteria.

Beware of the Snacks

Carol juggled a part-time job and two young children. She would take Toby to school and drop Sam off at the crèche before grabbing a large hot chocolate and an almond croissant from her favourite coffee shop on her way to work.

Carol would often work through her lunch break so she could get away early to run a few errands before collecting Sam and Toby at 3 p.m. To save time she would grab a bag of low-fat crisps and a reduced-fat chocolate bar to munch in the car. Preparing the children's tea inevitably meant she ate some of their chips and the odd leftover fish finger! Once the kids had finished eating, she would sit down with her partner Paul to enjoy their favourite cheesy bacon pasta bake.

Once Carol knew about the Carb Curfew diet plan she could see where she had been going wrong. She learnt how to make better choices on the run; how to read food labels effectively so she was no longer misled by 'reduced fat' labels, and how to have more nutritious snacks throughout the day.

Carol made some healthy adjustments to her daily diet: breakfast became a cappuccino, a bagel and a bottle of orange juice; for lunch she brought a thermos of soup from home, which she could have at her desk while she finished her work, or a pitta bread with carrot sticks and a small pot of cottage cheese; mid-afternoon she had a frozen banana smoothie, which she would make for herself and the boys; her evening meal became Lamb and Vegetable Hot-Pot (see page 168), or Lime Marinated Grilled Salmon with Salsa (see page 201) was another particular favourite, which she would serve with potatoes for Paul.

How did Carol do?
After 12 weeks Carol had lost 8 pounds of weight and her body fat had dropped from 36 per cent to 32 per cent, which meant she saw a considerable change in her body shape.

Watch Out for those Misleading Labels

As well as nutritional facts, food labels tell us about their contents by using terms such as 'low-fat' and 'sugar-free'. While this can be useful you should be aware that labels can be misleading. One food may be described on the label as 'low-fat' but in actual fact this may be a relative term used to describe the high-fat product against the 'lower fat version'. Mayonnaise is a classic example of this – individuals purchase the 'low-fat' version often thinking they are saving themselves lots of fat calories. This however is often a fallacy.

The information on food labels can help you compare the types and amount of fat in specific foods – which is very useful when a flash on the front of a box does not necessarily tell us the whole story. For example, peanut butter labels may read 'cholesterol free' – this is true but it never had cholesterol in it in the first place! Be wary not to fall into the trap of thinking that cholesterol-free means fat-free. Some cereal manufacturers claim 'no added fat' on muesli or wholesome cereal products, yet the natural grains have been processed with coconut or palm oils, which are high in saturated fat. So the answer is learn to look at the small print on the food labels and not just rely on the 'low-fat' or 'reduced-fat' label flashed on the front of the foods.

A Final Word

Don't worry if you feel you are a real fat-food junkie – with a little effort you can still enjoy your food and your desire for high-fat foods will decrease. Remember, this is not about cutting out all fat from the diet but rather reducing your overall fat intake, whilst at the same time increasing those good sources of fats. You can do this. Good luck!

Take Action

- ◎ Cut down on your intake of saturated and trans fats.
- ◎ Assess which is your most common source of saturated fat. For most people this will be cheese.

Depending on your personal attitude you may like to think about these courses of action:

a. cut out cheese for the next 7 days
b. reduce consumption
c. purchase lower fat alternatives

- Start reading your food labels.
- Look to maintain and even increase your consumption of foods high in essential fatty acids such as oily fish. Build up to three servings a week.
- Stop eating crisps and croissants.
- Consume no more than 40 grams of fat a day.
- For health purposes, fat intake should not fall below 10 grams a day.

chapter six

Be Consistent –
You Only Have to Be Good 80 Per Cent of the Time

How many times have you gone to bed on a Sunday night resolving that you will be really strict with yourself this week – you will say no to chocolate, sweets or naughty nibbles and you will go to the gym every morning before work? And how many times have you actually managed to achieve this? Of course this sort of do or die strategy never works. Even a handful of chips or a mouthful of chocolate will make us feel like we have failed. Such an extreme approach just sets us up to feel guilty and frustrated that we are unable to achieve our weight-loss goals.

The good news is this: the best way to lose weight, body fat and to stay healthy is not to deprive yourself of everything you love but instead to stick to the 80-20 rule. With the 80-20 rule, the key to successful long-term weight loss is consistency rather than being 'good' 100 per cent of the time. If you can stick to the Carb Curfew diet for just 80 per cent of the time you have succeeded! Yes it is true, being consistent means that you can actually eat a little more, you will feel more energetic, you will get the results you are seeking and the best bit is you stop setting yourself up for guilt and 'failure'.

So the final strategy in the Carb Curfew diet plan is to be consistent. In this chapter you'll learn why consistency is the key to successful long-term weight management and how to:

◎ Make the 80-20 rule work for you.
◎ Develop damage-limitation strategies that put you in control.

Carb Curfew Essentials

1. Stay within a sensible range of calorie and fat gram intake.
2. Get to know the triggers that prompt you to eat unwisely.

How Consistent Are You?

Answer the following questions to find out if you are prone to big swings in your food intake.

1. Do you overeat one day and then undereat the next in an attempt to save your calories?
2. If you have binged one day, do you starve yourself the next?
3. Do you have a history of dieting?
4. Do you go on extreme low-calorie diets and then go back to your 'normal' eating habits once you have lost some weight?
5. Do you experience plateauing with your weight?
6. Do you starve yourself to get into your favourite outfit for a special occasion?
7. Do you beat yourself up and think you have 'blown' your diet by having a chocolate biscuit or packet of crisps?

If you answered mostly yes, you are a classic erratic dieter. There are probably large variations in your calorie intake and you are likely to experience great fluctuations in your weight and body fat. In addition, you are probably prone to putting on weight very quickly, especially around times of excess such as Christmas and holidays. Psychologically, you may experience frustration at eating a low-calorie diet yet never being able to achieve your weight and body fat goals. You may also feel you are sometimes in a situation of free-fall with your weight, where whatever you try just keeps the scales moving up and not down. You probably also experience fluctuations in energy as you strive to keep your calorie content low one day only to find yourself completely devoid of energy the next and consequently needing to eat more.

Action: Focus first on achieving a Carb Curfew and decreasing your overall fat intake. These two simple steps will automatically help you to be more consistent in other areas.

If you answered mostly no, you are probably a fairly consistent eater who keeps their calorie and fat gram intake relatively stable. If you are still having trouble reaching your weight and body fat goals, you may need to have a close look at your diet to figure out which specific aspects of it are coming between you and your goals.

Action: Put the damage-limitation strategies into practice (see end of chapter for more about this). Identify what triggers you to eat unwisely, and use portion control and the starch-free zone.

Does This Story Sound Familiar?

Sue starts her week with great intentions: she eats very little on Monday – no breakfast, a coffee and a diet biscuit for lunch, and a low calorie ready-prepared meal for dinner. Sunday was a dieter's nightmare, she thinks, so she had better make up for all those extra calories she has eaten. She gets through Tuesday with the same determination, although she develops a bad headache from all the coffee she has been drinking to help her concentrate and curb her appetite. Wednesday comes and by 3 p.m. it's no good – the old vending machine calls and two bars of chocolate, a bag of crisps and a Danish pastry pass Sue's lips as hunger and lack of energy drive her to that instant sugar fix. In the evening she feels like she has blown her diet so she grabs some fish and chips on her way home from a few drinks after work. Thursday arrives and Sue still really wants to get into that new outfit she bought for the party on Friday night, so she says no to breakfast (better make up for the fish and chips she thinks), she grabs a slim shake at lunch and a low calorie can of soup for dinner. Friday comes so it's the obligatory no breakfast, can of low calorie soup for lunch and then off to the party. Well, she gets into the dress but she does not feel great, her energy levels are flagging and she feels quite nauseous from eating so little – the first glass of wine hits her very empty stomach … Sue starts Saturday feeling a little bit delicate so masses of toast and butter all round, lunch with friends, drinks in the evening, followed by the cinema with a box of chocolates! Sunday – well, tomorrow is Monday so she might as well enjoy herself today, ready for her 'diet' onslaught again. But this week she vows to be better.

The Verdict

If you actually counted out the amount of calories Sue consumed each day, you can see that even though her average daily calorie intake may be in the region of 1,500 calories – which is considered to be 'acceptable' for weight-loss purposes – her daily calorie intake has varied from 800 calories to in excess of 3,200 calories. This means that even though she may have consumed on average the right number of calories over the course of the week, she experienced great swings in energy, which culminated in her grabbing the quick sugar fix and not achieving an effective sensible weight loss. The weight Sue will have lost will have been from a loss of water and not a decrease in the size of her fat cells. Also, more importantly, Sue's actions are setting her up for long-term weight-loss failure. She will continually feel frustrated as she is depriving herself of food and important nutrients yet never making progress with her weight and body fat goals.

Sue needs to be more consistent – the best bit about being consistent is that it means she can actually eat a little more, feel more energetic, stop beating herself up and get the results she wants.

The 80-20 Rule

So as we have already established, the key to successful long-term weight and body fat loss is to apply the 80-20 rule. With the 80-20 rule you don't have to be 'good' 100 per cent of the time – you just need to be consistent and stick to the Carb Curfew diet plan for 80 per cent of the time and you will succeed.

Applying the 80-20 Rule

To apply the 80-20 rule, ideally you will keep your calorie and fat gram content down within a certain daily range. The calorie range for losing weight is between 1,200–1,500 calories per day depending upon how active you are. Applying this rule means you have a 500 calorie cushion each day. As you are also looking at the amount of fat grams in your diet, try and keep these within a range of 30–50 grams a day. If you consistently keep within these bands you will not only lose weight and body fat but more importantly for your health and happiness, you will keep the weight and body fat off. The longer you give your body the opportunity to burn the same range of calories and fat grams the more efficient it will become at using the calories from your food. Applying the 80-20 rule means that not only will you have more energy but also when you do overeat, your body will be able to use the extra calories more effectively rather than storing them in the fat cells.

Carb Curfew Tip

Aim to consume $3/5$ of your food by 5 p.m. – this will fuel you with energy during the day and help prevent you overeating in the evening when you are tired and your will power is at its lowest.

Carb Curfew Consistency Makeover

Anna works hard and plays hard. She is a busy 28-year-old executive who has a hectic social life and a demanding job. Before she embarked on the plan she was experiencing a lot of frustration with her weight despite going to the gym and following a 'diet'. So let's have a look at Anna's previous eating habits – here are three typical days in Anna's life:

Sunday
Breakfast: cup of herbal tea
Lunch: mushrooms fried in olive oil; 3 slices of soda bread; green salad with lettuce, tomatoes, peppers and rocket

Mid-afternoon snack: large packet of crisps
Dinner: low-fat tomato and basil soup; 3 slices of soda bread

Monday
Breakfast: cup of herbal tea
Lunch: large jacket potato with cottage cheese; small green salad with tomatoes and grated carrots
Mid-afternoon snack: cup of herbal tea
Dinner: bowl of low-fat tomato and basil soup; smoked mackerel salad; 3 slices of soda bread

Tuesday
Breakfast: fruit salad with pineapple, melon, apple and grapes; sesame seed bagel
Mid-morning: cappuccino and a croissant
Lunch: pasta, pesto and parmesan salad; low-fat chocolate and ginger muffin
Mid-afternoon snack: 2 chocolate biscuits; handful of little cheesy biscuits
Dinner: Thai restaurant meal shared between two – chicken satay, fish cakes, prawns, mussels, chicken drumstick, Pad Thai, boiled rice, green chicken curry, sizzling seafood platter; after-dinner mint; half bottle of red wine

Anna was a classic erratic. Her calorie and nutrient intake swung between extremes, leaving her devoid of energy and unable to reach her weight-loss targets. A look at

Anna's diet diary shows she ate roughly 1,200 calories on Monday compared to a whopping 3,500 calories on Tuesday. It's no surprise that by Wednesday morning Anna didn't feel like she had achieved much towards her diet goal. Anna's inconsistent eating meant she was nowhere near the 80-20 rule's 500 calorie cushion. Here is what Anna says:

'I felt such horror when I first started to record what I was eating. All the peaks and troughs in those figures were enough to put me off fat for life! When I started to put the 80-20 rule into practice and balance out my calorie and fat intake, I really began to feel the difference.'

Anna's Makeover Menu

Anna's makeover involved putting together a plan that fitted with her busy life. She needed to be more organized about her meals and a little thought soon paid huge dividends. Breakfast started to become a regular part of her daily meal plan and the Carb Curfew was a great success to help stabilize her overall calorie intake.

Breakfast: fruit smoothie – made from 250ml soya milk, a selection of fruit including a banana and one tablespoon of wheatgerm; a plain bagel
Mid-morning: piece of fruit

Lunch (from work canteen): rice and vegetable stir-fry, or chicken and salad stuffed tortilla, or pasta with a tomato-based sauce (large portion – Anna's own words!)
Mid-afternoon snack: yoghurt, or piece of fruit, or a shop-bought fruit smoothie
Dinner: salmon steaks with yoghurt and dill dressing with a green salad and tomatoes (no dressing)
Post-dinner: 6 almonds or piece of fruit

Anna's Verdict
So what did Anna really think about her makeover:

> *'The smoothies are great for breakfast – I really look forward to them and feel great because I know they give me a healthy start to my day. Introducing a Carb Curfew was obviously a huge change in my diet, but boy does it work! In general I now take a lot more care over my evening meal and I find I am eating a much more varied diet. And it really works well for me at home and with all my eating out at restaurants. I am enjoying cooking for myself and find it doesn't really take too much more effort to grill a piece of chicken or salmon than it does to boil a pan of water for pasta.*
>
> *To begin with I did find it a bit tough reducing my overall fat intake – especially giving up my chocolate biscuits and cheese – but the results speak for themselves. These days when I do eat "naughty food" I no longer feel too guilty and I certainly don't feel like*

*a failure. I know that my diet is sensible and the fact
that I have dropped nearly three dress sizes speaks for
itself. I feel fantastic!'*

So how did Anna do?
Over four months Anna dropped three dress sizes, she
lost three inches off her belly button and waist measurements, three inches off her hip and thigh measurements
and a total of fifteen pounds of body fat. Anna feels fitter
and healthier than she has done for a long time and she
certainly still lives her life to the full.

Never Eat on Two Feet!

How many times do you slip something into your mouth
without even realizing it? Maybe you are in the kitchen and
you are popping food into your mouth while you cook or you
are walking past a plate of biscuits or sweets and grabbing
a couple as you go – and before you know it you have
munched your way through 500 calories. And this is without
even sitting down and really appreciating your food. So to
help you avoid snacking make sure you always sit down to
eat. Remember the mantra: Never eat on two feet! You'll be
surprised what a difference it can make.

Does Your Lifestyle Trip You Up?

We have now learnt how to apply the 80-20 rule and seen how we can have a more relaxed approach to diet and fitness just so long as we are consistent. But in real life there will always be times when we cannot help going overboard – those big nights out, birthday celebrations, Christmas festivities and holidays, for starters. And on a day-to-day level there are also situations that lead us into temptation.

Everyone has different triggers that prompt them to overeat or eat all the wrong foods. Below are some common trigger activities, cues and locations – I am sure at least two or three of these are familiar to you. Identifying your triggers is a key step to achieving consistency and learning how to apply damage limitation to your diet plan.

Identifying Your Triggers

- boredom
- watching TV
- need a reward
- tired
- cold
- in the kitchen
- preparing food
- clearing food away

- social events
- birthdays
- feeling low and need to be cheered up
- feeding the children
- time of day
- menstrual cycle
- binge eating after a night on the town
- it's the weekend
- feeling frustrated at work
- eating out at restaurants
- 'I've been good all day so I'll treat myself'
- thinking you can overeat after exercise
- finishing chores so you feel you deserve a cup of tea and something to eat
- having a box of chocolates in the house knowing they are there waiting to be eaten
- being on holiday
- lonely
- long car journey
- food shopping when you are hungry
- losing your will power when drinking with friends
- friends who tempt you with goodies
- mid-afternoon
- biscuits at work
- comfort eating
- sugar cravings

So as you can see from the list above, there are lots of different situations that can act as triggers. We all have a different trigger profile – the challenge for you is to be honest with yourself and really get to know your own profile. Then you will be able to take charge of your triggers rather than your triggers taking charge of you.

You need to understand what prompts you to eat unwisely, whether this is overeating or selecting less healthy choices. Often your perception of a situation, a sequence of events or simply the time of day can act as a cue for you to either eat when you don't need to or to eat inappropriate foods. This I term 'head hunger'. By developing an understanding of the events that act as a trigger for you to eat inappropriately you can differentiate between 'head hunger' and 'genuine hunger'. You can then start to take control of your actions and develop eating patterns that not only help you reduce excess fat intake and calories but also keep your energy levels well fuelled.

Carb Curfew Tip

Stop beating yourself up – if you overindulge one day do not drastically deprive yourself and fast the next. Instead, eat a little less than normal and boost your usual activity level by having a really good workout at the gym or walking some of the way to work etc.

Damage-Limitation Strategies

If from time to time you know that your lifestyle isn't going to fit into your Carb Curfew diet plan, don't despair. The plan has built-in strategies that allow you to balance things out over time. Damage limitation means being realistic about your own habits.

When it is Difficult to Say 'No'

If you are following the Carb Curfew diet plan you will be trying to keep to a starch curfew. But some nights starch-free is just not possible. Perhaps you are going to eat at a friend's house and you know pasta is her favourite, or you are going to an Indian restaurant where unless you stick to salads, you most definitely will want some starchy rice or bread to mop up your lamb pasanda. Here are some damage-limitation suggestions to help you cope with a wide range of situations.

Option 1: Portion Control

If you are faced with a meal that is high in starches and fats, you can use portion control to make sure that all is not lost. Portion control allows you to enjoy high-calorie foods without having to worry too much about consuming excessive calories and fat grams. By making sure your portion size is limited, you can be assured that you have limited your calorie and fat gram intake without having had to say 'no', getting embarrassed or offending your hosts.

Portion control can be achieved by using a smaller plate than usual, by serving a smaller portion than you usually would take, or simply by not quite finishing the portion on your plate.

Option 2: Starch-Free Zone

On days when the Carb Curfew is out of the question – perhaps you know in advance that you will be eating starch at dinner – you can limit the damage done to your Carb Curfew diet plan by bringing in the starch-free zone.

The starch-free zone shouldn't be necessary too often but you will find it a useful support tool to your healthy eating plans. As I explained in chapter three, the starch-free zone means no bread, pasta, rice, potatoes or cereal in your midday meal. This then gives you the freedom to consume starch in your evening meal. It has all the benefits of the basic Carb Curfew but gives you the flexibility to accommodate an evening meal situation where you might not be able to go starch-free. Situations such as eating at friends' houses, a special buffet party, pancake day or maybe those times when you are eating out for both lunch and dinner, are all ideal times to apply the starch-free zone. Here are some examples of how to put the starch-free zone into practice:

Eating at a friend's home
Advice: go starch-free at lunchtime

A special buffet party
Advice: select starch-free options wherever possible. Have a fruit smoothie before going to party to curb appetite. Only allow yourself one trip to the buffet table

Eating in a restaurant for lunch and dinner
Advice: consider which venue it is easier to go starch-free – generally it is easier to do it at lunchtime as it limits any difficulties later. Have fruit for breakfast to help save some calories

Tips from Successful Carb Cutters

Paula
'Always keep in the car some sesame ryvita with half-fat cream cheese and of course a bottle of water. This will avoid you snacking on crisps and chocolate during long journeys.'

Lucy
'When I go to restaurants I find I overeat, especially when I look at the men sitting with me. Being only 5 foot 2 they are always much bigger than me. I always used to eat as much as them – now I watch what they eat and I aim to eat about 25 per cent less food than they do.'

Julie
'If you are prone to over-indulging on family comfort foods don't just put them away, cling wrap, seal, bolt or hide them! Do whatever you have to do to put a time and distance parameter between you and temptation. For example, a very effective strategy for me is to put food in the basement where the ironing is!'

A Final Word

Being consistent does not mean you have to wear your diet hat all the time. In fact, with the Carb Curfew diet plan you should feel in control to enjoy your food and achieve your weight and body fat goals. Remember, if you can stick to the plan for 80 per cent of the time you have succeeded! Knowing how to make damage limitation work for you will allow you to still live your life to the full and have fun with all the different situations that can get in the way of your good intentions. Keep going – you can make this work for you!

Take Action

◎ Make sure you keep to your Carb Curfew and remember the other nutritional strategies discussed earlier – and be consistent. Remember the 80-20 rule!

- ⊚ Identify the triggers that prompt you to eat unwisely so you can make healthier food choices in the future.
- ⊚ Plan ahead to identify those times when it may be hard to be consistent. If you are aware of these situations you can prepare yourself with the damage-limitation strategies.

chapter seven

Some Suggestions For Eating Out

Eating out in a restaurant is about relaxing and enjoying the food and company – you don't want to spend your evening worrying about what is on the menu because you are on a diet. This is where the Carb Curfew is different to a lot of other diets – it gives you the freedom to enjoy your meal, guilt free! By saying no to starches in your evening meal, you can relax and enjoy a wide range of other foods on the menu. Following are some suggestions of good dishes to choose when you are eating in a variety of restaurants – all the dishes listed are healthy and starch-free alternatives. You will probably be surprised to see just how much choice you have. I have also included some general tips for your midday meal.

I have not listed any suggestions for desserts – when you eat a dessert you pile on the extra calories without really needing them. Try waiting 20 minutes before saying yes to a sweet course to establish whether you are still truly hungry. If you decide you do want one, select fresh fruit and sorbets – they are the healthiest choices. Alternatively, opt for a peppermint tea to aid your digestion.

Remember, if you really know you are not going to be able to operate the Carb Curfew, you can always use the starch-free zone at lunchtime.

Italian

Although we tend to think that pasta and pizza dishes dominate an Italian menu, you can often find grilled chicken and fish on the menu – both are good choices either at lunchtime or in your evening meal.

If you are eating in an Italian restaurant at lunchtime, order a starter portion of pasta with a tomato-base rather than cream sauce or a small thin crust pizza. Avoid cheese and salami meat toppings on pizzas and say no to the garlic bread.

If you are eating Italian food in the evening, here are some good starch-free dishes to choose from the menu.

Starters:

Parma ham with figs or melon

Tomato and mozzarella salad (request without olive oil)

Tuna and bean salad

Gazpacho soup – although originally a Spanish dish you will often find this favourite on Italian menus

Main Courses:

Any grilled meat or poultry, for example, pollo cacciatore (chicken with tomato sauce) or vitello scallopine napoletana (veal with tomato sauce)

Any fish dish, for example, mixed fish salad or calamari

Indian

Spicy Indian meals can be a great choice because even a small portion can satisfy your taste buds! However, be careful because many dishes are full of fat. Go easy on the vegetable side dishes as they can be laden with ghee (clarified butter high in saturated fat), and select chicken or prawn dishes rather than beef or lamb dishes to save some calories.

If you are eating your midday meal in an Indian restaurant, remember that the starchy naan bread and rice accompaniments can boost unwanted calories. Select plain boiled rice rather than pilau rice and choose chappati as opposed to naan bread.

Here are some delicious starch-free dishes to choose for your evening meal.

Starters:
Cucumber raita
Chicken sashlik
Tomato sambal
Onion sambal
Mulligatawny soup

Main Courses:
Chicken tikka
Tandoori chicken
Tandoori king prawns
Tandoori mixed grill
Bhuna dishes baked with tomato and onions
Chicken jalfrezi
Vegetable curry

Thai

There are generally plenty of healthy choices on a Thai menu and the portions tend to be reasonably small. Thai salad dressings are great – often made with lime or lemon juice mixed with fish sauce and a little sugar. If eating chicken satay, go easy on the peanut sauce because it is laden with calories. Also, avoid coconut milk and all cream dishes.

If you are eating Thai food at lunchtime there are many delicious Thai spiced soups to enjoy which are made with stock and prawns or chicken with rice noodles and vegetables. These are filling and satisfying soups – and the addition of the starchy noodles fuels you with energy for the afternoon.

If you are eating in a Thai restaurant in the evening, here are some good starch-free dishes to choose:

Starters:
Tom yam gung (hot and sour soup with prawns)
Gai tom ke (chicken, coconut and galangal soup)

Main Courses:
Thai beef salad
Yam talay (tasty seafood salad)
Pla manow (fish with lemon sauce)
Normai pad kai (pork with bamboo shoots)
Moo pad king (pork with ginger)

English

Ask anyone to name a couple of typical English dishes and steak and kidney pies and spongy puddings will probably pop into their mind – not great dishes if you are trying to say no to starches. With a little care however it is possible to navigate your way around the menu and eat very healthily and happily.

For lunch, choose an open sandwich instead of the traditional closed sandwiches – a great combination is a slice of wholemeal bread spread with a little cranberry sauce, topped with a pile of salad greens, grated carrot and a grilled chicken breast or chicken or turkey slices. If grabbing something from a café opt for a ham roll (and eat only one piece of the roll) rather than a cheese and tomato sandwich. A poached egg on toast with a couple of grilled tomatoes is another great way to get a good balance of starch and protein at lunchtime.

Here are some delicious suggestions for your evening meal:

Starters:
Soup – but steer clear of creamy varieties. Say no to the bread roll that accompanies it
Smoked salmon – say no to the bread and eat with salad garnish
Prawn cocktail with a little dressing

Main Courses:
Select roast chicken and turkey rather than cuts of beef, lamb and pork. Remember not to eat the skin

Select casseroles such as venison in red wine, chicken with vegetables and pork and apple. Say no to the potatoes and ask for extra vegetables

Grilled gammon steak with pineapple and salad – make sure you cut off the visible fat before you eat it

Chargrilled salmon with salad – ask for it not to be served drenched in butter

American

The main challenge of eating out US-style is the size of the portions. This is where portion control really comes in. So although offers such as 'eat all you like' can be a good deal, in terms of the Carb Curfew diet plan you are going to have to assert a little self discipline!

Everyone (except those who are vegetarian) loves burgers and a small hamburger (no cheese, no mayonnaise) with a salad garnish contains just 250 calories, so you don't have to say no to burgers at lunchtime. It is when you start adding all the extras that the story changes. American restaurants do great soup and salad bars at lunch times – they also do great dressings and they love to put loads of sauces, dips and dressings on all their dishes. So 'help-yourself' salad bars can be great but watch out for the creamy dressings, bacon pieces, croutons and grated cheese. Instead, enjoy the crunchy vegetables such as carrots, broccoli and celery, pile up your plate with water-dense vegetables such as tomatoes, lettuce and cucumber, and enjoy a little olive oil dressing.

Here are some starch-free suggestions for your evening meal:

Starters:
Vegetable crudités with salsa dip
Mixed salad
A spicy virgin bloody mary – this will satisfy your taste buds and curb your appetite
Corn on the cob (request no butter)
Vegetable soup

Main Courses:
All steaks: rump, fillet and sirloin contain less than 325 calories per 240g portion. Eat with salad but chop off the visible fat
Burgers (say no to the bun) and eat with extra relish and salad toppings
Roast quarter chicken (no skin)
Chargrilled jerk chicken salad
Cajun grilled prawns with spinach salad

Chinese

Traditional Chinese cuisine is low in fat but be careful when eating Chinese food from commercial restaurants and takeaways – a lot of the food is deep fried or cooked in excess oil and this can really add on calories. Also, the monosodium glutamate can make you feel bloated and thirsty after your meal as well as the following day. Remember, you can ask to have your food prepared without the MSG.

I am a big fan of soups for lunch – they are filling, nourishing and can be eaten on the run. Bean curd broth is an excellent health choice and won ton soup (chicken and dumplings) is great if you want something a little more substantial. If you feel like something other than soup, prawn or chicken chop suey is a good lunchtime choice.

If you are eating Chinese food in the evening, here are some delicious starch-free suggestions:

Starters:
Hot and sour soup
Crab and sweetcorn soup
Chicken noodle soup
Chicken and sweetcorn soup

Main Courses:
Chicken and stir-fried vegetables
Steamed vegetables
Pork and pineapple
Steamed bok choi (green cabbage) in oyster sauce
Tofu and steamed vegetables
Steamed fish with ginger and spring onion
Chicken and black bean sauce
King prawns with Chinese vegetables

Greek

Grilled meat and fish and delicious low-calorie vegetables such as tomatoes, aubergines, peppers and olives tend to form the base of Greek food. However, be careful of the amount of olive oil you are consuming as often these dishes arrive swimming in the stuff. While good for the heart remember it still contributes to the calories.

A lunchtime snack of taramaslata and pitta bread may seem appealing but be careful how much you eat – taramaslata is laden with hidden fat. It is better to choose dolmades (stuffed vine leaves) or select one of the starter suggestions below. My favourite is a small Greek salad with grilled sardines and a small pitta bread. If you fancy something lighter try the avgolemono (chicken and lemon soup).

Here are some good starch-free suggestions for your evening meal:

Starters:
Olives
Hummus
Grilled sardines
Avgolemono
Tzatziki (natural yoghurt with cucumber and mint)

Main Courses:
Marinated calamari (drain off the oil)
Keftedes (meatballs)
Traditional Greek feta cheese salad – but ask for the olive oil dressing on the side
Grilled lamb and pepper kebab
Fish baked in tomato sauce
Kleftiko (very slow roasted lamb on bone)
Souvlakia (lamb grilled on skewers)

French

When eating French-style watch out for the butter, oil and cream – and of course the customary basket of baguettes. Remember, you can always ask them not to bring the bread to the table if you know you will find it hard to resist.

Instead of opting for a croque monsieur at lunchtime try a lobster bisque or bouillabaisse (fish soup) with a side salad or a starter portion of moules marinière. Traditional moules marinière is mussels cooked with dry white wine, onion, garlic, parsley and thyme, but some restaurants add cream so check first and ask for it without. The added bonus of moules is the time it takes to navigate the shells will give your stomach time to tell you when it is full!

If you are eating French food in the evening, here are some tasty starch-free dishes to choose from the menu.

Starters:
French onion soup
Salade nicoise (leave the potatoes and ask for the dressing on the side)
Bouillabaisse – say no to the bread spread with rouille
Lobster bisque

Main Courses:
Grilled dover sole or trout
Steak tartare
Moules marinière
Ratatouille
Chicken chasseur
Salmon in red wine
Coq au vin
Steak au poivre

Japanese

Traditional Japanese food is based on fish, raw vegetables, noodles and rice – with very little meat – and is renowned for being healthy. The fish is often served raw and if you have not tried it, you will probably be surprised at how tasty it is.

Japanese cuisine is becoming increasingly popular at lunchtime instead of our traditional sandwich. Sushi boxes can now be found in most supermarkets and sandwich bars and they make a tasty lunch, offering a good balance of protein and starch as well as being naturally low in saturated fat and calories. You will find them a great way to satisfy you and fuel you with energy for the afternoon.

For your evening meal you can enjoy teppan dishes which are cooked on a griddle, or why not try raw or steamed tofu or sashimi, which is raw fish accompanied by grated white cabbage.

chapter eight

Carb Curfew Recipes

This chapter is full of ideas for your Carb Curfew meals when eating at home, showing you how easy it can be to incorporate the Carb Curfew diet into your life. Maybe you just want to cook a quick meal for yourself, or you have a hungry family to feed, or you have invited some friends over for dinner – whatever the occasion, you will find a recipe to suit it. Following is a collection of meat, fish and vegetarian recipes for lunchtime and your evening meal. All the recipes are low in fat and calories and provide you with the right balance of nutrients at the right time of the day. The emphasis of Carb Curfew cooking is on healthy dishes that are easy to cook as well as appetizing and enjoyable to eat.

Be Prepared

Before you begin cooking it is important to be prepared. You need to make sure you have a sufficiently stocked storecupboard so you have the right ingredients on hand when you need them.

Your Carb Curfew storecupboard should always contain a variety of grains and starch sources such as bread, cereal, rice and pasta – this will provide you with a good range of nutrients and dietary fibres. Porridge oats should be a staple item in your storecupboard – when you eat porridge at breakfast it provides you with a great source of slow energy releasing carbohydrates which set you up for the day. Wheatgerm is another highly nutritious ingredient that is a must-have in your Carb Curfew kitchen – it can be added to smoothies or used to top cereals as well as being an ingredient in its own right.

Fruit and Vegetables

Don't worry if you don't always manage to buy fresh fruit and vegetables – just make sure you have tins of fruit (in natural fruit juice) and vegetables (preferably in water with no added sugar or salt) on hand. It is best to buy water-dense fruit and vegetables such as spinach, cucumbers, tomatoes, peppers, strawberries and melons as they are low in calories and they can help to hydrate you. Frozen fruit and vegetables are very useful to store in the freezer – as we have already seen, frozen fruit makes a great addition to smoothies. Next time you are in your local supermarket, check out the frozen fruit and veg aisle. And remember, you can always freeze your overripe bananas – peel and cut into chunks, place in small freezer bags and pop in the freezer for use at a later date.

Dried Fruit

Dried fruit is naturally low in fat, a good source of dietary fibre and iron, and it can give you a good natural sugar energy boost – but beware of the calories. A 50g bag of pineapple, papaya or mango provides 270 calories and a 50g bag of apricots provides 165 calories – so buy little individual bags to avoid a big bag of dried apricots suddenly disappearing in one go!

Dairy Products

When buying dairy products, always select the low-fat varieties wherever possible. Fromage frais, for example, is a great low-fat alternative to yoghurt. Also, get into the habit of buying organic soya milk and organic tofu. Both tofu and soya milk are low in calories and highly nutritious; they are also good sources of phyto-oestrogens, which have been shown to have a protective effect against some reproductive cancers.

Meat, Fish and Poultry

When buying your fresh meat, fish and poultry buy in bulk and then freeze in smaller portions for convenience – this works particularly well with chicken breasts and fish fillets. And don't forget about canned sources of fish like pilchards, sardines, pink salmon and tuna, which can make handy economical protein sources for lunch and supper. They are also an excellent source of omega-3 essential fats: remember the Carb Curfew diet plan is not about cutting out all fat from your diet – rather it is about consuming the right types of fats. Pre-cut wafer thin sandwich meats are also great to have on hand for snacks. Try lean ham, chicken and turkey for the lowest calorie value and saturated fat content.

Pulses and Beans

Pulses such as butter beans, chick peas and kidney beans are a key ingredient in the Carb Curfew diet – especially if you are a vegetarian – so stock up on them. They provide an excellent source of dietary fibre as well as being good sources of minerals and B-complex vitamins; they also help control blood sugar levels and lower blood cholesterol levels. You can either buy pulses dried or in cans – dried pulses need soaking for anything up to five hours, so if you are short of time you may prefer to use the canned variety.

Seeds and Nuts

Your storecupboard should also always contain seeds and nuts, which are an excellent source of protein. Nuts can add a great crunch element to your diet and they provide an excellent source of vitamin E as well as other minerals and vitamins including vitamin B. But beware – these healthy additions to your diet have a high calorie content: 100g of cashews, pistachios, almonds or hazelnuts contain over 550 calories and more than 45g of fat. So be careful how many nuts you nibble! Seeds such as linseeds, sesame, sunflower and pumpkin are excellent sources of essential fats. Linseeds, for example, are great added to smoothies, porridge and casseroles – crush them with a pestle and mortar to release their beneficial health properties.

Oils and Vinegars

Monounsaturated oils such as olive oil are a better choice to cook with than polyunsaturated oils as they are more stable when heated at higher temperatures. Polyunsaturated cold-pressed oils such as flax seed oil (found in the fridge section of health-food shops) are not stable when heated so do not use for cooking. Instead, keep in the fridge and use as a dressing on salads. Don't overlook flavoured vinegars as they can add a variety of tastes to low-fat dressings, marinades and seasonings. If you are able to invest in good-quality vinegars your taste buds will really notice the difference.

Miscellaneous

While the aim of the Carb Curfew diet is to limit the use of additional sugar in your cooking, all storecupboards will contain some sugar. You may wish to use an artificial sweetener such as aspartame to keep your calorie content down. But beware – some studies have shown that a high intake of these artificial sweeteners can cause additional carbohydrate cravings and have harmful effects on health. So you may prefer to use the natural thing – but use sparingly! Natural fruit spreads and fresh honeycomb are preferable over commercial high-sugar jams.

Finally, don't forget to stock up on fresh herbs. Buy pots of herbs from your supermarket, pop them on your window ledge and let them grow. As you will see from the following recipes, they are a must-have ingredient in the Carb Curfew storecupboard.

Carb Curfew Lunches

Here is a selection of recipes for your midday meal, which provide a good balance of starch and protein. Some you will find work better to eat at home – others can easily be put in a lunch box to go. By omitting some of the starch accompaniments you can also double these up as Carb Curfew dinners.

At the end of each recipe you will see the calorie and fat content per serving.

Mexican-Style Wraps with Beans, Herbs and Vegetables

SERVES 1

100g canned kidney beans
100g canned asparagus
2 tablespoons plain fromage frais
1–2 tablespoons coriander leaves
1 tablespoon flat-leaf parsley
1 tablespoon finely chopped red onion
1 tablespoon lime juice
1 plum tomato
1 soft flour tortilla
salt and pepper, to taste

In separate sieves, drain the kidney beans and asparagus thoroughly. In a mixing bowl, mash the asparagus until smooth. Stir in the fromage frais, coriander, parsley, onion and lime juice. Season to taste with salt and pepper and set aside.

Quarter the tomato and scoop out the seeds. Cut the flesh into small pieces and fold into the asparagus mixture along with the kidney beans.

Lay a tortilla out on a work surface and spread with the vegetable mixture. Fold over a portion of the left-hand side of the tortilla then roll up from bottom to top to give a cylinder. Eat immediately or wrap in greaseproof paper or kitchen foil and pack in a lunch box.

calories per serving: 293   *fat grams per serving: 10*

Vegetables Menestra

SERVES 2

150g fresh or frozen peas
150g fresh or frozen broad beans
150g asparagus
1 teaspoon olive oil
1 garlic clove, chopped
25g Serrano ham, chopped
1 teaspoon flour
3 canned artichokes, halved
1 tablespoon chopped fresh parsley

To serve:
Slice of fresh rye or pumpernickel bread or a small baked potato

Bring a large saucepan of water to the boil. Add the peas, broad beans and trimmed asparagus, return to the boil and simmer for 3 minutes until the vegetables are cooked but still quite crisp. Drain well.

Heat the oil in a large frying pan and add the chopped garlic. Cook over a medium-low heat, stirring constantly, until the garlic is just golden. Add the ham and cook, stirring, for about 3 minutes, then stir in the flour and cook for another 2–3 minutes.

Stir in the cooked vegetables and artichokes and cook, while stirring, for another 3 minutes until the vegetables are tender and the artichokes are heated through. Transfer to a bowl and sprinkle with the chopped parsley. Serve accompanied by fresh bread or a baked potato, if desired.

calories per serving: 204   fat grams per serving: 4

Smoked Chicken and Mexican Black Bean Salad

SERVES 1

150g cooked black beans
40g smoked chicken or turkey
60g red pepper
30g celery, any leaves reserved
15g spring onion
10g fresh coriander
1 teaspoon finely chopped green chilli
juice of 1 lime
salt and pepper, to taste

To serve:
Slice of toasted granary bread

Place the black beans in a mixing bowl. Cut the smoked chicken or turkey into strips and stir it into the beans. Finely dice the pepper, celery and spring onion and stir them in too.

Roughly chop the reserved celery leaves with the leaves and tender stalks of the coriander. Stir them into the salad with the green chilli. Pour in the lime juice and season to taste with salt and pepper. Transfer to a serving plate or lunch box. Serve with toasted granary bread.

calories per serving: 260   fat grams per serving: 3

Salmon Pizza

SERVES 1

75g fresh salmon fillet or 200g can pink salmon, boned and
   skinned
1 small pizza base
1–2 tablespoons fresh tomato sauce
1 tomato
1 tablespoon chopped red onion
½ teaspoon dried red chilli flakes (optional)
3 tablespoons low-fat yoghurt
1 sprig fresh dill

Preheat the oven to 220°C/425°F/Gas mark 7. Trim the
salmon of any skin and bones and dice the flesh. Place the
pizza base on a baking tray and spread with the tomato sauce.
Dice the tomato and sprinkle it over the sauce, then sprinkle
with the red onion and chilli flakes. Arrange the diced salmon
evenly over the top.

   Bake for 15–20 minutes or until the fish is cooked and the
pizza base is lightly browned. Remove from the oven, spoon
on the yoghurt and garnish with fronds from the sprig of dill.

calories per serving: 365   fat grams per serving: 18

Salmon, Potato and Asparagus Salad

SERVES 2

1 large salmon fillet
3 stalks asparagus
150g baby new potatoes
½ mango
50g low-fat yoghurt
½ teaspoon wholegrain mustard
1 tablespoon lemon juice or white wine vinegar
1 tablespoon chopped fresh chives
½ stick celery
140g mixed salad leaves
salt and pepper, to taste

Place the salmon in a shallow pan and cover with water. Bring to the boil, then throw in the asparagus, cover and turn off the heat. Leave to stand until the cooking water reaches room temperature.

Meanwhile, place the potatoes in a large saucepan, cover generously with water and bring to the boil. Lower the heat and simmer for 10 minutes until tender. Drain, refresh under cold running water and set aside to cool.

Chop the mango and combine in a blender with the yoghurt, mustard and lemon juice or vinegar. Process until smooth, then stir in the chives by hand. Season to taste with salt and pepper and place the dressing in the fridge to chill.

Remove the salmon and asparagus from the poaching liquid and pat dry with kitchen paper. Cut both into bite-sized pieces and place in a bowl with the cooled cooked potatoes.

Chop the celery finely and add it to the bowl. Gently fold in the mango-yoghurt dressing.

Arrange the mixed salad leaves in a salad bowl, top with the dressed salmon and vegetables and serve.

calories per serving: 285   fat grams per serving: 13

Pasta with Spring Vegetables

SERVES 1

100g dried pasta such as penne
1 teaspoon vegetable bouillon powder
50g asparagus spears
50g baby carrots, or sliced regular carrots
50g baby courgettes, or sliced regular courgettes
50g mangetout or fine beans, trimmed
1 teaspoon balsamic vinegar
15g parmesan cheese, shaved
2 teaspoon shredded basil leaves
1 teaspoon finely chopped green part of spring onion
freshly ground black pepper

Bring a large saucepan of water to the boil. Add the vegetable bouillon powder and stir to dissolve. Add the pasta and cook according to the directions on the packet. Leave the pasta to boil while you prepare the vegetables, trimming and slicing them as necessary.

Five minutes before the end of the pasta's cooking time, add the asparagus, carrots, courgettes and mangetout or beans – do not stir. Continue cooking for 5 minutes or until the pasta and vegetables are all al dente. Drain thoroughly.

Place the pasta and vegetables on a serving plate and sprinkle with the balsamic vinegar. Top with the shavings of parmesan, the basil and spring onion. Grind some black pepper over the top and serve.

calories per serving: 229   *fat grams per serving: 7*

Carb Curfew Dinners

Here is a selection of starch-free recipes for your evening meal. You'll find something for every occasion be it a family dinner, a simple meal for two or a dinner party. The emphasis of the dishes is on protein, essential fats, low-fat dairy products and vegetables. All Carb Curfew dinners also work well as starch-free zone lunches.

At the end of each recipe you will see the calorie and fat content per serving.

Meat Dishes
Lamb and Vegetable Hot-Pot

SERVES 4

200g onions
200g carrots
200g swede or turnip
200g parsnip
1 tablespoon vegetable oil
500g cubed lamb stewing steak
340ml bitter beer (large can)
1 bay leaf or bouquet garni
salt and pepper

Preheat the oven to 150°C/300°F/Gas mark 2. Peel all the vegetables and cut them into bite-sized pieces. In a large non-stick frying pan, heat the oil and add the cubed lamb. Cook over a high heat, stirring frequently until the meat is brown on the outside but not cooked through. Transfer to an oven-proof lidded casserole dish.

Add the vegetable pieces to the frying pan, working in batches if necessary, and cook until just beginning to brown. Transfer the vegetables to the casserole and stir well. Pour in the beer, then add the bay leaf or bouquet garni and season generously with salt and pepper. Cover the casserole and place in the oven for 2 hours. Halfway through the cooking time remove the lid and stir. The hot-pot is done when the meat and vegetables are very tender and most of the beer has been absorbed. Remove the bay leaf or bouquet garni and season again to taste before serving.

calories per serving: 424   *fat grams per serving: 15*

Grilled Steaks with Asparagus and Balsamic Shallots

SERVES 2

2 lean beef steaks
2 garlic cloves
200g shallots
4 tablespoons balsamic vinegar
1 crumpled bay leaf
1 teaspoon olive oil
200g asparagus
1 teaspoon flaked sea salt, plus extra to season
freshly ground black pepper

Preheat the oven to 180°C/350°F/Gas mark 4. Place the steaks in a non-corrosive dish. Crush the garlic finely and rub it over the steaks. Season generously with sea salt and pepper and set aside to marinate for 30–60 minutes.

Peel the shallots and trim the ends. Halve lengthways and place in a small oven-proof dish in which the shallots fit snugly – this is important. In a small bowl, combine the balsamic vinegar with 100ml of water and pour it over the shallots. Add the bay leaf and place in the preheated oven for 30 minutes.

Meanwhile, place the olive oil in another oven-proof dish and add the trimmed asparagus. Rub the asparagus with the oil then sprinkle with the sea salt and black pepper. When the shallots have been cooking for 30 minutes, remove them from the oven and stir thoroughly. Return the shallots to the oven, placing the dish of asparagus in the oven at the same time and cook for another 20 minutes.

Ten minutes before the end of cooking the asparagus and shallots, heat a griddle over a very high heat until smoking. Use kitchen paper to wipe the crushed garlic from the steaks, then add them to the pan. Immediately turn the heat down to medium-low and cook for 1–2 minutes on each side, depending on how thoroughly you like steak cooked.

Remove the shallots and asparagus from the oven and arrange on serving plates. Top with the steak and serve accompanied by a chutney or mustard, if desired.

calories per serving: 268   fat grams per serving: 16

Thai Beef Salad

SERVES 2

For the beef:
2 lean beef steaks
juice of 1 lime
1 tablespoon soy sauce

For the salad:
150g tomatoes
100g celery
100g spring onions
100g carrot
15g coriander

For the dressing:
1–2 small red chillies
1 garlic clove
1 teaspoon fish sauce
1/2 teaspoon palm sugar, brown sugar or honey

Place the steaks in a non-corrosive dish. Set aside 2 table-spoons of the lime juice in a small bowl and pour the remainder over the steaks. Add the soy sauce to the meat and set aside to marinate for 30–60 minutes.

Meanwhile, make the salad. Using a small knife, score a cross in the base of each tomato. Place them in a heat-proof bowl and cover with boiling water. Leave to stand for 1–2 minutes, then drain and refresh under cold water. When cool, peel and core the tomatoes. Discard the seeds and cut the flesh into strips. De-string the celery and cut into matchsticks. Cut the spring onions into fine strips. Use a vegetable peeler to cut the carrot into ribbons. Combine the vegetables in a salad bowl. Roughly chop the coriander, including the tender stalks, and stir it into the vegetables.

To make the salad dressing, crush the chillies and garlic together using a pestle and mortar to make a paste. Stir in the reserved 2 tablespoons of lime juice, plus the fish sauce and sugar or honey.

Heat a griddle over a very high heat for about 5 minutes or until very hot and smoking. Add the marinated steaks and immediately turn the heat down to medium-low. Cook for 1–2 minutes on each side, depending on how thoroughly you like steak cooked.

Pour the salad dressing over the vegetables and toss well. Place the vegetables on serving plates and top with the cooked steak – you can cut the steak into strips first if you prefer.

calories per serving: 444   *fat grams per serving: 19*

Spicy Sausage with Cherry Tomato Sauce and Broccoli Chilli Pesto

Sausages are generally a high-fat food but here is a recipe that uses storecupboard ingredients and the family-favourite sausage to achieve a Carb Curfew dinner. Serve with a salad and you have a well-balanced and tasty evening meal.

SERVES 2

250g spicy Italian fresh sausages

For the cherry tomato sauce:
1 teaspoon olive oil
300g cherry tomatoes
paprika or cayenne pepper, to taste

For the broccoli chilli pesto:
stem of 1 head broccoli
3–4 basil leaves
1–2 green olives
½ teaspoon dried chilli flakes
salt and pepper, to taste

To make the broccoli chilli pesto, chop the broccoli stem into small pieces. Place in a small saucepan, cover with water and bring to the boil. Simmer for 5–8 minutes or until the broccoli stem is very tender. Drain well, reserving the cooking water, and allow to cool briefly.

Transfer the broccoli to a food processor or blender and add the basil, olives, chilli flakes and a little salt and pepper.

Process until smooth, adding just enough of the reserved cooking water to make a spoonable paste. Adjust the seasonings to taste and set aside.

Now make the cherry tomato sauce. Place the olive oil in a large heavy-based saucepan. Rinse the cherry tomatoes and add them to the pan without letting them dry. Cover the pan and set over a low heat. Cook for about 3 minutes, shaking the pan frequently. Remove the lid and mash the cherry tomatoes a little with a wooden spoon – the mixture should form a sauce but retain some texture. Add the paprika or cayenne, cover the pan again and continue cooking gently for another 5–10 minutes, stirring occasionally.

Meanwhile, preheat the grill to the highest setting. Cook the spicy sausages on a rack set over the grill pan so that the excess fat drains away during cooking. Turn frequently during cooking – the exact time needed will depend on the thickness of the sausages.

Adjust the seasonings of the cherry tomato sauce to taste, then arrange a pool of sauce on the serving plates. Top with the cooked sausages, then add a dollop of the broccoli chilli pesto.

calories per serving: 536   *fat grams per serving: 44*

Renee's Chargrilled Lamb

SERVES 2

2 x 150g lean lamb steaks

For the marinade:
1 small glass red wine
2 tablespoons soy sauce
1/2 tablespoon chopped fresh thyme
1/2 tablespoon chopped fresh mint
1/2 tablespoon chopped fresh tarragon
1/2 tablespoon chopped fresh rosemary

Mix together all the ingredients for the marinade.

Trim any excess fat from the lamb steaks and place them in a bowl with the marinade, making sure they are well coated. Place in the fridge and leave to marinate for at least 2 hours or overnight.

To cook, grill or barbecue the lamb, basting occasionally. Cook for 5–10 minutes, depending on how pink you like your meat to be. Serve with a nice green salad.

calories per serving: 333   *fat grams per serving: 12*

Gammon Steaks with Thai-Style Salsa

SERVES 2

2 x 125g gammon steaks
Vegetable oil spray

For the salsa:
100g tomatoes
100g cucumber
100g carrots
50g celery
50g spring onions
1 tablespoon chopped fresh coriander
6 tablespoons lime or lemon juice
1–2 teaspoons fish sauce or soy sauce, to taste
4 tablespoons mild sweet chilli sauce

First make the salsa. Chop all the vegetables very finely and place in a bowl. Stir in the remaining ingredients and set aside to marinate while you cook the gammon steaks.

Heat a griddle or heavy-based frying pan over a very high heat. Spritz the pan with vegetable oil spray, then lay the gammon steaks in the pan and lower the heat to medium. Cook for about 3 minutes on each side until nicely browned and hot.

Serve the gammon steaks immediately with the salsa.

calories per serving: 291   fat grams per serving: 10

Italian Calves' Liver with Carrot and Fennel Salad

SERVES 2

250g calves' liver
2 teaspoons plain flour
25g bacon
200g onions
2 teaspoons olive oil
2 tablespoons red or white wine vinegar
salt and pepper, to taste

For the salad:
150g carrots
100g fennel bulb
juice of 1/2 lemon
1 teaspoon olive oil
1 tablespoon fresh coriander leaves

To serve:
1 tablespoon chopped fresh parsley

Cut the liver into strips and place in a plastic bag. Add the flour, seal and shake gently until the meat is evenly coated. Chop the bacon and onions into small dice.

Heat the olive oil in a large non-stick frying pan. Fry the bacon and onions, stirring frequently, for about 10 minutes until the onion is very soft and golden. Remove the mixture from the pan with a slotted spoon and set aside on a plate in a warm place.

178

Remove the liver from the plastic bag, add the meat to the pan and cook over a medium heat, turning frequently, until it is done. Return the onion mixture to the pan, add the vinegar and season with salt and pepper. Bring to a simmer then lower the heat right down and keep warm while you make the salad.

Grate the carrots and finely dice the fennel bulb. Combine in a salad bowl with the lemon juice, olive oil and coriander leaves. Season to taste with salt and pepper and toss well.

Serve the salad with the liver and onion mixture, sprinkled with the chopped fresh parsley.

calories per serving: 347   fat grams per serving: 13

Marinated Oriental Pork Fillet with Sweet and Sour Vegetables

SERVES 2

4 x 115g pieces pork fillet

For the marinade:
4 tablespoons balsamic vinegar
2 tablespoons clear honey
2 garlic cloves, crushed
1/2 teaspoon wasabi paste (optional)

For the vegetables:
8 small bok choi or 1/2 head Chinese leaf
50ml rice wine or dry sherry
1 teaspoon soy sauce
1/2 teaspoon ground ginger
8 small shallots
2 small carrots, diagonally sliced
1 courgette, diagonally sliced
2 celery sticks, diagonally sliced
1 teaspoon sesame oil
salt and freshly ground pepper, to taste
coriander sprigs, to garnish

For the sauce:
1 lemon grass stalk
1 bay leaf
100ml rice wine or dry sherry

50ml white wine vinegar
$^1/2$ teaspoon light soy sauce
200ml tomato juice
200ml pineapple juice

Blend all the marinade ingredients in a non-metallic dish. Add the pork, turn to coat, cover and chill for at least 2 hours.

Preheat the oven to 190°C/375°F/Gas mark 5.

Blanch the bok choi in a pan of boiling water for $1^1/2$ minutes, drain and refresh under cold water. Drain and squeeze out any excess water. Lay the bok choi in a large shallow ovenproof dish, pour over the rice wine or sherry and the soy sauce, and sprinkle over the ginger. Cover tightly and bake for 20 minutes.

Heat a sturdy roasting tin to hot on the hob. Remove the pork from the marinade, place in the roasting tin and sear for 2–3 minutes until lightly browned all over, then roast in the oven for about 15 minutes until cooked through.

Meanwhile, heat a large heavy-based non-stick frying pan over a high heat. Add the shallots and cook for 1 minute. Add the remaining vegetables, cook for 3–4 minutes, then stir in the oil and season to taste. Fry for 2 minutes more until the vegetables are charred. Keep warm.

To make the sauce, place the lemon grass, bay leaf, rice wine or sherry, vinegar and soy sauce in a small pan and boil over a high heat until reduced by two-thirds. Add the fruit juices and reduce by a further two-thirds, then pass through a fine sieve. Keep warm.

Arrange the charred vegetables and bok choi on serving plates, drizzle over the sauce and top with the pork. Garnish with fresh coriander.

calories per serving: 335   *fat grams per serving: 9*

Chicken Dishes
Chicken and Apricot Tagine

SERVES 4

8 skinless, boneless chicken thighs
150g dried apricots, chopped
225g onions, chopped
225g mushrooms, chopped
725ml chicken or vegetable stock
a pinch of saffron
a pinch of ginger
a pinch of cumin
salt and pepper, to taste
fresh coriander to garnish (optional)

Place all the ingredients in a large, heavy-based saucepan or casserole dish and bring to the boil. Cover, lower the heat right down and simmer for 45 minutes, stirring occasionally.

When cooked, remove the lid and simmer uncovered until most of the liquid evaporates and you have a thick stew. Adjust the seasoning to taste and serve garnished with fresh coriander if desired.

calories per serving: 259   fat grams per serving: 5

Chilled Chicken Salad with Smoked Paprika

SERVES 2

For the chicken:
2 skinless, boneless chicken breasts
vegetable stock or water to cover
a splash of vinegar, white wine or lemon juice
1 bay leaf or bouquet garni

For the salad:
2 red peppers
75g cucumber, sliced or chopped
140g mixed salad leaves
2–3 tablespoons fresh parsley leaves

For the sauce:
125g plain low-fat yoghurt
2 teaspoons sun-dried tomato paste
1½–2 tablespoons finely chopped fresh herbs such as basil,
    chives, parsley
1 small garlic clove, crushed
1 tablespoon lemon juice
⅛–¼ teaspoon smoked paprika, or to taste
salt and pepper, to taste

Place the chicken breasts in a frying pan with the vinegar, white wine or lemon juice and the bay leaf or bouquet garni. Cover with vegetable stock or water and bring to the boil.

Lower the heat to a very gentle simmer and cook for 25 minutes until the chicken is done.

Meanwhile, start preparing the salad. Heat the grill to the highest setting and grill the red peppers whole until they are blistered and blackened all over. Remove from the heat, place in a bowl and cover with clingfilm. Leave to stand for 10 minutes to make the skins easier to remove.

When the chicken is cooked, remove it from the pan and set aside to cool on paper towels. Peel the black skin from the peppers, discard the core and seeds and cut the flesh into strips. Combine in a salad bowl with the cucumber, salad leaves and parsley.

In a small mixing bowl, combine all the ingredients for the sauce. Cube the cooled chicken and stir it into the sauce. Arrange the salad on serving plates, top with the dressed chicken and serve.

calories per serving: 251   fat grams per serving: 6

Light Chicken Curry with Spinach

SERVES 2

2 medium-large onions, finely chopped
500ml chicken or vegetable stock
1 large Bramley or other cooking apple, peeled, cored and diced
1 tablespoon sultanas
1 heaped tablespoon garam masala
2 part-boned chicken breasts
140g baby spinach leaves
fresh coriander to garnish
salt and pepper, to taste
a little freshly grated nutmeg (optional)

Place the onions and half the stock in a casserole dish or heavy-based saucepan and bring to a hard boil. Lower the heat, cover and leave to simmer for 15 minutes until the onions are tender. Remove the lid and raise the heat a little. Simmer until the liquid has almost evaporated, then add the apples and sultanas and cook for 5 minutes, stirring occasionally. Add the garam masala and stir to give a thick sauce, then add the chicken and stir until thoroughly coated with the sauce. Pour in the remaining stock and bring to the boil. Cover and lower the heat right down so that the stew simmers very gently for 30 minutes.

Uncover the stew and remove the cooked chicken to a plate. Raise the heat under the pan and simmer until the sauce mixture has reduced to a thick coating consistency. Return the chicken to the pan and add salt and pepper to taste. Allow to heat through briefly.

Meanwhile, place the washed spinach in a large saucepan over a low heat. Cover and cook for 5 minutes, stirring occasionally, until the leaves have wilted. Add salt and pepper to taste, plus some grated nutmeg if desired.

Divide the spinach between the serving plates. Top with the chicken and sauce and garnish with the fresh coriander.

calories per serving: 402   *fat grams per serving: 9*

Provencal-Style Poached Chicken with Vegetables

SERVES 2

2 skinless, boneless chicken breasts
725ml chicken stock
4 tablespoons white wine
1 teaspoon herbes de Provence mixture
100g tomatoes
100g broccoli florets
100g courgettes
75g leeks
75g baby carrots
1 tablespoon finely chopped fresh parsley, to garnish
salt and pepper, to taste

Place the chicken breasts in a frying pan with the stock, wine and herbes de Provence. Bring to the boil, then cover and simmer gently for 20 minutes.

Meanwhile, put a kettle of water on to boil. Using a small knife, cut a small cross in the base of the tomatoes. Place in a heat-proof bowl and cover with the boiling water. Leave to stand for 1–2 minutes, then drain and peel the tomatoes. Discard the seeds, reserving as much of the tomato juice as possible. Cut the flesh into strips and set aside with the juices.

Cut the broccoli, courgettes and leeks into bite-sized pieces. When the chicken has been cooking for 20 minutes, add all the vegetables including the tomato strips and carrots, then season to taste with salt and pepper. Cover and cook for another 5 minutes or until the chicken is fully cooked and the vegetables are just tender.

Transfer the vegetables and chicken to large soup bowls and top with a generous quantity of the broth. Sprinkle with the parsley and serve with knives, forks and soup spoons so that diners can enjoy the broth.

calories per serving: 174   *fat grams per serving: 4*

Swedish Chicken and Apple Salad

SERVES 2

For the salad:
175g ready cooked chicken breast, diced
1 small dessert apple, cored and sliced
1 carrot, coarsely grated
2 spring onions, sliced
15g walnut pieces, chopped
1 small head chicory leaves
salt and freshly ground black pepper, to taste
salad cress, to garnish

For the dressing:
100ml low-fat plain yoghurt
1/2 teaspoon mild curry paste
1 tablespoon fresh lemon juice
1 small garlic clove, crushed
1/2 teaspoon sugar
3 tablespoons freshly chopped herbs (eg. parsley, mint and dill)
salt and freshly ground black pepper, to taste

Blend all the dressing ingredients together in a small bowl. Add the diced chicken, sliced apple, carrot, spring onions and walnuts. Season well. Mix together and then chill for 30 minutes.

To serve, line a serving platter with the chicory leaves and pile the salad on top. Scatter the salad cress over the dish and serve.

calories per serving: 292   fat grams per serving: 9

Honey and Orange Chicken with Chilli Vegetable Salad

SERVES 2

For the chicken:
4 x 110g chicken thigh fillets, skinned and de-boned
2 teaspoons curry powder
1 teaspoon cornflour
125ml orange juice
1 tablespoon lemon juice
1 tablespoon honey
2 teaspoons mustard
salt and pepper

For the chilli vegetable salad:
200g broccoli florets
100g cauliflower florets
100g carrots, thickly sliced
2 tablespoons mild sweet chilli sauce
1 tablespoon soy sauce
2 teaspoons lime juice
1 tablespoon chopped fresh coriander
Freshly ground black pepper

Preheat the oven to 180°C/350°F/Gas mark 4. Skin and trim the chicken thighs, as necessary. Place in a plastic bag with the curry powder, cornflour and some salt and pepper. Seal the top of the bag and shake until the chicken pieces are evenly coated with the curry powder mixture.

In a jug, mix together the orange and lemon juices, honey and mustard and some salt and pepper. Remove the chicken pieces from the bag, place them in a small ovenproof dish and pour the orange-honey mixture over the top. Turn the chicken pieces to coat thoroughly, then place in the oven for 45 minutes. Turn and baste halfway through cooking.

Meanwhile, boil the broccoli, cauliflower and carrots for 5–8 minutes or until tender but still with some bite. Drain and refresh under cold running water, then drain again thoroughly.

In a salad bowl, combine the chilli sauce, soy sauce, lime juice and coriander, adding black pepper to taste. Add the drained vegetables and toss. Serve at room temperature with the glazed baked chicken.

calories per serving: 399   *fat grams per serving: 13*

Cajun Chicken with Red Pepper Salsa

SERVES 2

For the chicken:
2 x 125g chicken breasts, skin removed
Pinch crushed dried chilli or chilli powder (more if you like it firey)
1 teaspoon paprika
1/2 teaspoon ground coriander
1/2 teaspoon ground cumin
Pinch garlic salt

For the salsa:
1 small red chilli, deseeded and finely chopped
1 red pepper, deseeded and finely chopped
4 plum tomatoes, skinned, deseeded and finely chopped (you could
    use canned tomatoes for convenience)
1 garlic clove, crushed
2 teaspoons olive oil
juice of 1 lime
freshly ground black pepper

Slice each chicken breast in half across the middle. Combine the dried chilli or chilli powder, paprika, coriander, cumin and garlic salt and mix well. Rub the seasoning onto the chicken and marinate for 2 hours.

Mix all the salsa ingredients together and leave for 2 hours.

Grill the chicken under a medium heat for about 15 minutes, turning frequently and let the Cajun seasoning slightly blacken prior to serving. Spoon the salsa over the chicken and serve with a green salad or steamed broccoli and fennel.

calories per serving: 346   *fat grams per serving: 15*

Bangers and Root Vegetable Mash

SERVES 2

250g low-fat chicken or turkey sausages

For the root vegetable mash:
200g celeriac, peeled and diced
200g carrots, peeled and diced
2 tablespoons low-fat plain fromage frais
freshly grated nutmeg, to taste
salt and pepper, to taste

For the gravy:
1/2 teaspoon cornflour
2 tablespoons white wine or sherry
100ml chicken stock
2 teaspoons chopped parsley
1 teaspoon Worcestershire sauce, or to taste

To serve:
100g savoy cabbage

Heat the oven to 180°C/350°F/Gas mark 4. Separate the sausages, put them in an ovenproof dish or roasting tin and place in the oven. Bake for 30–40 minutes until cooked through and golden brown. Turn twice during cooking to help ensure even browning.

Meanwhile, make the root vegetable mash. Place the celeriac and carrots in a saucepan of salted water and boil for about 20 minutes until very tender. Drain and mash thoroughly. Beat the fromage frais into the mash until smooth, then season with the nutmeg and salt and pepper. Set aside in a warm place until ready to serve.

Now make the gravy. Mix the cornflour into the wine or sherry and place the mixture in a small saucepan with the stock, parsley and Worcestershire sauce. Bring to the boil and stir constantly for 2–3 minutes until the sauce just thickens. Season with salt and pepper as necessary. Remove from the direct heat and set aside in a warm place until ready to serve.

Shred the cabbage finely and steam or boil it for 5 minutes in a small saucepan. Serve hot with the cooked sausages, gravy and root vegetable mash.

calories per serving: 298   fat grams per serving: 7

Stir-Fried Chicken in Black Bean Sauce

SERVES 2

For the stir-fry:
250g cubed chicken
2 teaspoons cornflour
100g red pepper
100g shallots or mild onion
100g mangetout
50g celery
1 teaspoon vegetable oil
50g bean sprouts
160g bottle ready-made black bean sauce

To serve:
few sprigs of fresh coriander
1 spring onion, finely chopped

Place the chicken in a plastic bag. Add the cornflour, seal and shake until the chicken is evenly coated. Set aside while you prepare the vegetables.

Cut the red pepper into bite-size chunks. Cut the shallots or onion into fine wedges. Trim the mangetout at each end and cut in half crossways. Slice the celery into 1cm pieces on the diagonal.

Heat the vegetable oil in a wok or large non-stick frying pan. Add the chicken and stir-fry for about 5 minutes until cooked. Using a slotted spoon, remove from the pan to a large plate or bowl.

Add the pepper and shallots to the pan and stir-fry for 2–3 minutes until cooked but still crunchy. Remove from the pan and add to the chicken. Add the mangetout and celery to the pan and sir-fry for 2–3 minutes until just starting to soften.

Pour the black bean sauce into the pan and add the bean sprouts. Bring to simmering point, stirring often, and then return the cooked chicken and vegetables to the pan. Heat through for 3 minutes, then serve garnished with the chopped spring onion and sprigs of coriander.

calories per serving: 558   fat grams per serving: 14

Fish Dishes
Grilled Tuna with Beetroot Hummus

SERVES 2

For the fish:
2 small tuna steaks
1 tablespoon Thai sweet chilli sauce
1 teaspoon sesame oil

For the beetroot hummus:
250g cooked beetroot
400g canned chickpeas
1 teaspoon cumin
1–2 cloves garlic
juice of 1 lemon
1 teaspoon sesame oil
salt and pepper, to taste

For the salad:
100g watercress or rocket leaves
50g salad onions or scallions, finely sliced

Place the tuna in a non-corrosive dish and rub with the chilli sauce and sesame oil. Leave to stand in a cool place for 1–2 hours to marinate.

Meanwhile, place all the ingredients for the hummus in a blender and process to a slightly textured paste. Add just enough water to give the mixture the consistency of thick yoghurt.

When ready to cook the fish, heat a griddle or heavy non-stick frying pan over a high heat until almost smoking. Add the fish and immediately lower the heat to medium-low. Cook the fish for 2 minutes on each side or until done to your liking. Alternatively, cook under an overhead grill heated to high.

Spoon the beetroot hummus onto serving plates and arrange the watercress or rocket and the salad onions next to it. Top the hummus with the tuna and serve.

calories per serving: 467   fat grams per serving: 13

Lime Marinated Grilled Salmon with Salsa

SERVES 2

For the fish:
2 small fillets salmon or other oily fish
grated zest and juice of 1 lime
2 teaspoons brown sugar
2 teaspoons olive oil
salt and pepper

For the salsa:
250g red pepper
250g tomatoes
50g mild onion
1 fresh green chilli
1 garlic clove, crushed
1–2 tablespoons fresh lime juice
1–2 tablespoons chopped fresh coriander leaves

Place the salmon in a non-corrosive dish. In a small bowl, combine the lime zest and juice, sugar, olive oil and salt and pepper to taste. Pour over the fish and leave to marinate for at least 30 minutes in a cool place.

Meanwhile, heat the grill to the highest setting. Place the peppers and tomatoes under the grill and cook until blistered and blackened all over, turning frequently. Remove each vegetable from the heat as it is done and transfer to a bowl and cover with clingfilm. Leave to stand for 10 minutes to make the skins easier to remove.

Peel, seed and core the peppers and tomatoes, reserving as many of the tasty juices as possible. Chop the flesh finely and place in a clean bowl with the juices. Finely chop the onion and green chilli and stir them into the salsa, along with the garlic, lime juice and coriander. Season to taste with salt and pepper.

When ready to cook the fish, heat the grill to high and remove the fish from the marinade, discarding the excess marinade. Cook the fish for 2–3 minutes on each side or until done to your liking. Remove from the heat and serve with the salsa.

calories per serving: 425   *fat grams per serving: 22*

Prawn, Scallop and Parma Ham Kebabs with Parsley Salad

SERVES 4

For the kebabs:
8 raw king prawns
8 fresh king scallops
2 garlic cloves, crushed
2 tablespoons chopped fresh basil
juice of 1/2 lemon
1 tablespoon olive oil
12 slices Parma ham or prosciutto crudo

For the salad:
150g fresh parsley
30g pitted black olives
4 spring onions
1/2 red onion
1 tablespoon lime or lemon juice
salt and pepper
300g tomatoes, thickly sliced
200g cucumber, thickly sliced

Remove the shells from the prawns, then clean and de-vein. Clean the scallops. Place the prawns and scallops in a non-corrosive bowl with the garlic, basil, lemon juice and olive oil. Add some salt and pepper and set aside to marinate for 15–20 minutes.

Meanwhile, make the salad. Chop the parsley roughly, discarding any coarse stems but retaining the tender ones. Place in a salad bowl. Very finely chop the olives, spring onions and red onion and stir them into the parsley, adding the lime or lemon juice and salt and pepper to taste.

Heat the grill to the highest setting. Gather a slice of ham into a ruffle and thread it onto a metal skewer. Then thread on a scallop and a prawn. Repeat and finish the kebab with another ruffle of ham. Prepare another three metal skewers the same way.

Place the kebabs under the grill and cook for about 5 minutes, turning and basting with the excess marinade frequently. They are ready when the ham is crisp and the shellfish is just cooked.

Meanwhile, lay the slices of tomato and cucumber in a circle on the serving plates. Top each with a mound of parsley salad, then lay a cooked kebab on top. Pour the cooking juices from the grill pan over the plate as a dressing for the salad.

calories per serving: 206   *fat grams per serving: 10*

Spiced Fish with Cajun Vegetables

SERVES 2

For the spiced fish:
1 large garlic clove
1/2 teaspoon fennel seeds
1/2 teaspoon black peppercorns
1/2 teaspoon dried mixed herbs
1/4 teaspoon cayenne pepper or paprika
a large pinch of salt
1 tablespoon cornmeal
2 skinned halibut fillets
1 tablespoon olive oil

For the Cajun vegetables:
1 green pepper, deseeded
1 small onion
1 stick celery
400g canned chopped tomatoes
1 bay leaf
1 teaspoon cayenne pepper or paprika
1/2–1 teaspoon molasses or black treacle, or to taste
salt and pepper, to taste

To prepare the Cajun vegetables, finely chop the green pepper, onion and celery. Place them in a heavy saucepan with the canned chopped tomatoes, bay leaf, cayenne or paprika, and molasses or black treacle. Add about 4 tablespoons of water and bring the mixture to the boil, stirring. Season to taste with salt and pepper. Cover the pan, then lower the heat right down and simmer gently for 20 minutes.

Begin preparing the spiced fish – use a pestle and mortar to crush the garlic, fennel and peppercorns until fine. Stir in the dried mixed herbs, cayenne or paprika, salt and cornmeal.

When the vegetables have been cooking for 20 minutes, remove the lid and allow to simmer uncovered, stirring constantly, until the mixture is thick and the excess liquid has evaporated. Set aside in a warm place.

Use the spice mixture to coat the fish evenly, pressing it into the flesh. Heat the olive oil in a frying pan over a high heat and cook the coated fish for 90 seconds on each side, or until lightly browned and cooked through.

Divide the vegetable mixture between the plates and serve the fish on top.

calories per serving: 360   *fat grams per serving: 15*

Salmon, Cannellini and Lemon-Infused Stew

SERVES 2

225g salmon fillet, skinned and cut into 2.5cm cubes
2 lemons
1/2 tablespoon olive oil
1 small onion, finely chopped
1 celery stick, finely chopped
2 bay leaves
227g can tomatoes
275ml vegetable stock
salt and pepper, to taste
227g can cannellini beans
chopped fresh parsley to garnish

Grate the rind of one lemon and shred a few strips from the other. Squeeze the juice of both and put aside.

Heat the oil in a large pan, add the onion and celery and fry for 10 minutes until softened. Stir in the bay leaves, tomatoes and stock. Season and simmer, uncovered, for 20 minutes.

Stir in the lemon juice and grated lemon rind, beans and salmon. Simmer for 8–10 minutes until the salmon is cooked. Spoon the stew into bowls and garnish with the lemon-rind strips and parsley.

calories per serving: 314   fat grams per serving: 13

Grilled Hake with Mushroom and Sweetcorn Sauce

SERVES 2

2 x 150g hake fillets (haddock, cod or skate works well too)
1 heaped teaspoon cornflour
140ml fish stock
20ml low-fat double cream
50g button mushrooms, finely sliced
2 egg yolks
1 small can sweetcorn, drained
olive oil spray
chopped fresh dill, to garnish

Mix the cornflour with a little water to make a smooth paste. Stir into the fish stock on a low heat and add the cream.

Dry-fry the sliced mushrooms. Gently heat the egg yolks in a bowl immersed in a pan of boiling water, adding a few drops of water as needed to create a smooth paste. Stir this into the fish stock and then add the mushrooms and sweetcorn.

Spray the fish with the olive oil and grill for about 5 minutes until brown, turning regularly.

To serve, place the fish on serving plates, top with the sauce and garnish with dill. This dish is lovely served with a fresh green salad.

calories per serving: 362   *fat grams per serving: 11*

Poached Oriental Seabass with Cucumber, Ginger and Spring Onion

SERVES 4

4 x 100g seabass fillets
1 teaspoon coconut milk
25g enoki (strand) or baby button mushrooms
1/2 teaspoon sesame oil
1 tablespoon lime juice
6 sprigs fresh coriander
2 tablespoons soy sauce
salt and freshly ground black pepper

For the garnish:
15g ginger, shredded
25g spring onion, shredded
25g cucumber, shredded

Place the coconut milk, mushrooms, sesame oil, lime juice, coriander and soy sauce in a shallow pan with 900ml of water. Bring to a simmer without a lid.

Season the fish and place in the water; poach gently. Remove the fish and keep warm. Increase the heat and reduce the poaching liquid by half. Pour the liquid over the fish and garnish with the remaining ingredients.

calories per serving: 168   fat grams per serving: 5

Lemon and Bay Fish Parcels with Roast Tomatoes

SERVES 2

2 x 150g fillets cod or other firm white fish

For the fish parcels:
150g fennel bulb, finely shredded
100g red or yellow pepper, diced
2 spring onions, chopped
1 lemon, finely sliced
6 bay leaves
2 tablespoons white wine
salt and black pepper

For the tomatoes:
150g vine ripened tomatoes
Olive oil spray
salt and black pepper

Preheat the oven to 180°C/350°F/Gas mark 4. Take two large squares of kitchen foil or greaseproof paper and divide the fennel, diced pepper, spring onions, lemon slices and bay leaves between them, making a pile of the vegetables in the centre of each sheet.

Lay the fish on top of each of the vegetable piles. Sprinkle a teaspoon of white wine and some salt and pepper over each. Fold up the parcels to enclose all the fish and the vegetables and then place them on a baking tray.

On a separate baking tray, place the tomatoes (halved if large) and spritz them lightly with olive oil spray. Sprinkle with a little salt and pepper to taste. Place both trays in the oven and cook for 15 minutes.

To serve, place a parcel on each serving plate and arrange the roast tomatoes on the side. (Don't forget to tell your guests to discard the bay leaves and lemon slices before eating.)

calories per serving: 164   *fat grams per serving: 3*

Vegetarian Dishes
Steamed Tofu and Aubergines with Aromatic Chinese Sauce

SERVES 2

220g plain or smoked tofu
200g aubergine
100g asparagus
100g broccoli

For the sauce:
2 tablespoons soy sauce
2 teaspoons oyster-flavoured sauce
2 teaspoons chilli sauce
2 teaspoons sesame oil
2 spring onions, chopped

Cut the tofu into equal-sized cubes. Finely slice the aubergine and cut the asparagus and broccoli into bite-sized pieces. Fill a saucepan with water to a depth of about 2¹/₂ cm and place a steamer over the top. Bring the water to the boil. Lay the tofu in the steamer and surround it with the aubergine, broccoli and asparagus. Cover and steam for 5 minutes.

In a small saucepan, combine the soy sauce, oyster sauce, chilli sauce and sesame oil. Bring to the boil and simmer for 2–3 minutes or until the mixture has thickened slightly.

Use a fish slice to transfer the cooked tofu and vegetables to serving plates. Pour the hot sauce over the top and garnish with the chopped spring onions.

calories per serving: 127   *fat grams per serving: 11*

Vegetable and Miso Soup with Teriyaki Tofu

SERVES 2

For the tofu:
220g tofu
2 tablespoons teriyaki marinade

For the soup:
100g carrot
100g cauliflower
100g broccoli
100g cabbage
400ml vegetable stock
1 tablespoon mirin or sherry
2 tablespoons miso
1 small chilli, sliced
2 spring onions, sliced
1 teaspoon sesame seeds

Cut the tofu into equal-sized blocks and rub with the teriyaki marinade. Place in a non-corrosive dish and set aside to marinate for 20 minutes.

Dice the carrot. Cut the cauliflower and broccoli into bite-sized pieces. Shred the cabbage. Place the vegetable stock and mirin or sherry in a large saucepan and bring to the boil. Add the chopped vegetables, stir and simmer for 5 minutes or until the vegetables are cooked.

Remove a ladle of broth from the pot and place in a small bowl. Stir the miso into the bowl of broth, then stir the miso and broth into the soup. Lower the heat under the pan right down – enough to keep the soup warm without letting it boil.

Heat a griddle or non-stick frying pan over a high heat until smoking. Lay the marinated tofu in the pan and immediately turn the heat down to medium-low. Cook for 2 minutes on each side, turning carefully with a fish slice.

Divide the soup between the serving bowls ensuring each diner has a mixture of vegetables. Top with the cooked tofu, then sprinkle with sliced chilli, chopped spring onions and sesame seeds. Serve hot.

calories per serving: 163   fat grams per serving: 7

Mexican Bean Chilli

SERVES 4

150g black beans
2 dried chipotle chillies
800g canned chopped tomatoes
1 red pepper
1 stick celery
1 small carrot
2 garlic cloves
1 teaspoon cumin
salt and pepper, to taste
2–3 sprigs fresh coriander

The day before serving, place the black beans in a bowl and cover generously with around 300ml water. Leave to soak overnight.

The next day, drain the black beans. Place in a saucepan and cover with around 300ml of fresh water. Bring to the boil and simmer for 1 hour or until the beans are tender – the exact time will depend on the age of the beans.

Meanwhile, in a small, heavy-based frying pan, toast the dried chillies over a very low heat until fragrant, turning frequently. Transfer to a small bowl. Pour 300ml of boiling water over the toasted chillies and leave to soak for 20 minutes. Remove the chillies from the soaking liquid and remove the cores and seeds. Chop the chillies roughly then return them to the soaking water. Using a hand blender, purée the chillies and soaking water together to give a hot, smoky liquid.

Place the chilli purée in a large saucepan and add the canned tomatoes. Chop the pepper, celery and carrot finely and add them to the tomato mixture. Crush the garlic and stir it in along with the cumin.

When the beans are tender, drain them and transfer to the tomato mixture. Bring the mixture to a boil, then lower the heat and simmer for 30 minutes or until the chilli is thick and all the flavours have amalgamated. Season to taste with salt and pepper. Serve garnished with the sprigs of fresh coriander.

calories per serving: 100   *fat grams per serving: 3*

Bean Burgers with a Light Caesar-Style Salad

SERVES 2

For the bean burgers:
150g cooked or canned black beans or other cooked beans
2 heaped tablespoons finely grated carrot
2 heaped tablespoons finely grated onion
2 tablespoons chopped fresh coriander
salt and pepper, to taste
1 teaspoon olive oil

For the salad dressing:
4 tablespoons low-fat yoghurt
3 tablespoons grated parmesan cheese
6 drops Tabasco sauce
6 drops Worcestershire sauce
1/4 teaspoon mustard
1/2 small garlic clove, crushed
1/4 teaspoon black olive paste or 1 anchovy

For the salad:
200g cucumber
250g mixed salad leaves

In a small bowl, mash the beans for the burgers thoroughly. Stir in the carrot, onion and coriander and season to taste with salt and pepper. Shape the mixture into 2 large burgers.

To make the salad dressing, combine the yoghurt, parmesan, Tabasco, Worcestershire sauce, mustard and crushed garlic in a bowl. If using black olive paste, stir it into the dressing; if using anchovy, rinse it thoroughly, pat dry and mince finely before stirring it into the dressing.

To cook the bean burgers, heat the oil in a non-stick frying pan. Place the burgers in the pan and immediately turn the heat down to medium-low. Cook for 2–3 minutes on each side or until crusty and golden brown on the outside. Transfer to a plate lined with paper towels to drain off oil and set aside in a warm place.

Halve the cucumber lengthways and scoop out the seeds using a teaspoon. Cut the flesh into bite-sized pieces and toss in a salad bowl with the mixed salad leaves. Drizzle the dressing over the top. Arrange the dressed salad on serving plates and top with the bean burgers. Serve the bean burgers warm.

calories per serving: 450   *fat grams per serving: 23*

Spanish White Bean Stew

SERVES 2

800g cooked or canned white beans such as cannellini or
    butter beans
1 large green pepper
1 large onion
1 large tomato
1 large carrot
1 red or green chilli
vegetable stock, to cover
2 teaspoons olive oil
salt and pepper, to taste

Finely dice all the vegetables. Place in a large saucepan with
the drained beans. Stir, then add enough vegetable stock to
cover the ingredients. Bring to the boil over a high heat, then
lower the heat right down and cover. Simmer for 30 minutes
or until the stew is soft, stirring occasionally. Season to taste
with salt and pepper. Divide amongst serving bowls and drizzle each bowl with 1 teaspoon olive oil before serving.

calories per serving: 383   *fat grams per serving: 8*

Lentil Loaf with Yellow Pepper Sauce

SERVES **4**

For the loaf:
125g green lentils
125g yellow split peas
125g chopped onion
1 egg
3 tablespoons olive oil, plus extra for greasing
2 tablespoons chopped fresh parsley
1 tablespoon chopped fresh tarragon
1 large garlic clove
$1/2$ teaspoon baking powder
$1/2$ teaspoon salt

For the sauce:
100g tomatoes
4 yellow peppers
1 tablespoon chopped basil
2 teaspoons white wine vinegar or sherry vinegar
salt and pepper, to taste

To make the lentil loaf, soak the green lentils and yellow split peas in a generous quantity of water for 4–5 hours or overnight. When ready to cook, preheat the oven to 190°C/375°F/Gas mark 5 and line a loaf tin with kitchen foil, greasing it lightly with olive oil.

Place all the ingredients for the loaf in a food processor and whizz until smooth and combined. Stir by hand halfway through if necessary to help move the ingredients around the bowl of the processor. Pour the lentil mixture into the prepared loaf tin and smooth over the top. Bake in the oven for 45–50 minutes.

Meanwhile, make the sauce. Put a kettle of water on to boil. Use a small sharp knife to cut a cross in the base of the tomatoes and place them in a heat-proof bowl. Cover with the boiling water and leave to stand for 1–2 minutes. Drain and refresh with cold water. When cool, peel and core the tomatoes. Discard the seeds but retain as many juices as possible. Cut the flesh into fine strips and set aside with the juices in a bowl.

Halve, core and deseed the peppers. Place them skin-side up on a foil-lined grill pan and grill for 20 minutes until the skins are black and blistered. Remove the pan from the heat and fold the foil up around the peppers to make a pouch. Leave to stand for 5 minutes so that the skins are easier to remove.

Peel the peppers, discarding the black skins, and transfer the flesh to a blender. Add the vinegar, basil and 1 tablespoon of water and process until smooth. Add more water as necessary to give the consistency of a thick sauce. Transfer the mixture to a small saucepan and add salt and pepper to taste. Heat through gently, then stir in the reserved tomatoes and their juices and keep warm until the lentil loaf is cooked.

Remove the loaf from the oven and cut into slices. Serve with the vegetable sauce poured over the top.

calories per serving: 270   fat grams per serving: 18

Asparagus, Pepper and Courgette Omelette

SERVES 4

2 onions
1 swede
1 carrot
2 teaspoons olive oil
300g canned asparagus
1 courgette
1 red pepper
125g reduced-fat Cheddar cheese
4 whole eggs plus 4 egg whites
salt and pepper, to taste

To serve:
200g mixed lettuce leaves
a squeeze of lemon juice

Preheat the oven to 180°C/350°F/Gas mark 4. Finely slice the onions, swede and carrot. Arrange in a large round oven-proof dish, preferably non-stick, and pour over the oil. Season lightly with salt and pepper. Cover with kitchen foil and bake for 30 minutes until tender.

Drain the asparagus thoroughly. Cut the courgette and pepper into sticks a similar size to the asparagus. In a mixing bowl, beat together the whole eggs and egg whites and season lightly with salt and pepper. Gently stir in the cheese.

Remove the dish of vegetables from the oven and remove the foil. Leave the oven on. Arrange the asparagus, courgette and pepper on top of the cooked vegetables like the spokes of a wheel. Pour over the egg mixture and bake uncovered for 15 minutes. Serve at room temperature with green salad leaves dressed with a squeeze of lemon and a little salt and pepper.

calories per serving: 266   *fat grams per serving: 17*

Pumpkin and Mushroom Stew

SERVES 4

1 large pumpkin, about 30cm diameter
200g onions
200g mushrooms
2 tablespoons olive oil
300ml vegetable stock
6 tablespoons flaked almonds or pine kernels
3 tablespoons low-fat fromage frais
2 tablespoons chopped fresh parsley
salt and pepper, to taste

Peel, core and deseed the pumpkin. Cut the flesh into bite-size pieces. Slice the onions and mushrooms. Heat the oil in a very large saucepan. Add the onions and stir-fry until golden. Add the pumpkin and continue cooking, stirring frequently, until it begins to brown. Add the mushrooms and cook until they begin to soften. Pour the vegetable stock into the pan, bring to the boil, then lower the heat and simmer until the pumpkin is tender and the cooking liquid has evaporated.

Meanwhile, in a dry frying pan, toast the almonds or pine kernels over a moderate heat, stirring frequently, until golden brown. Remove to a plate to cool.

When the pumpkin is tender, remove the pan from the heat and stir in the fromage frais and parsley. Generously season to taste and serve scattered with the toasted nuts.

calories per serving: 348   fat grams per serving: 30

Cheesey Baked Bean Hot-Pot

SERVES 2

450g can baked beans in tomato sauce
225g can chopped tomatoes
100g green or red pepper, finely chopped
2 teaspoons ready-made crispy onions
2 teaspoons chopped chives
2 tablespoons vegetarian Worcestershire-style sauce or brown sauce
20g grated low-fat Cheddar cheese
100g spinach leaves
pinch grated nutmeg
salt and pepper, to taste

In a small saucepan, place the baked beans, pepper, crispy onions, chives, Worcestershire sauce and cheese. Heat gently, stirring frequently, until the cheese has melted and the other ingredients are hot and tender. Season to taste.

Meanwhile, rinse the spinach leaves, shake dry and put them in a large saucepan with a pinch of salt. Cover and cook over a moderate heat for 3–5 minutes until the spinach has wilted.

Remove the lid, raise the heat and add the nutmeg. Cook, stirring often, until the juices have evaporated from the pan and the spinach is relatively dry. Season to taste. Arrange a bed of spinach on a serving plate and top with the cheesey baked beans.

calories per serving: 279   *fat grams per serving: 6*

Dijon Spinach Salad

SERVES 2

100g Fakin' Bacon, bacon-style Quorn or tempeh
100g cucumber
100g carrots
75g baby spinach leaves
25g mixed herb leaves (eg. basil, chives, dill, marjoram, parsley, watercress)
100g canned kidney beans, rinsed and drained
100g cherry tomatoes
1 tablespoon olive oil

For the dressing:
1 teaspoon olive oil
2 tablespoons white or red wine vinegar
2 tablespoons lemon juice
1 teaspoon Dijon mustard
salt and pepper

Cut the cucumber and carrots into ribbons or small bite-size pieces and combine in a large salad bowl with the spinach, herbs, kidney beans and cherry tomatoes. Toss thoroughly.

Cut the Fakin' Bacon, Quorn or tempeh into bite-size pieces. Heat the olive oil in a frying pan and add the Fakin' Bacon, Quorn or tempeh. Cook, turning occasionally, until golden. Remove from the pan and add to the salad bowl.

To make the dressing, add the olive oil, vinegar, lemon juice and mustard to the hot pan and stir vigorously with a wooden spoon over high heat to incorporate the caramelized cooking juices. Season to taste with salt and pepper.

Pour the hot dressing over the salad, toss and serve immediately.

calories per serving: 299   *fat grams per serving: 17*

Vegetable Frittata with Roasted Tomato Salsa

SERVES **4**

For the frittata:
olive oil cooking spray
4 shallots, sliced
100g mushrooms, sliced
450g tofu
2 egg whites
pinch sea salt
pinch ground white pepper
2 teaspoons granulated onion powder
large handful fresh basil, chopped
75g fresh spinach, blanched (boiled in water for 30 seconds),
   chopped
75g mozzarella cheese, grated

For the salsa sauce:
Olive oil cooking spray
2 large cans chopped tomatoes
2 large onions, chopped
1 shallot, peeled
pinch sea salt
fresh basil, chopped, to taste

Preheat the oven to 180°C/350°F/Gas mark 4. First prepare the frittata. Spray a heavy sauté pan with olive oil, and heat. Add the shallots and cook for 2 minutes, stirring constantly. Add the mushrooms, sauté for about 2 minutes until the mushrooms turn soft, then set aside to cool.

In a food processor, purée the tofu and gradually add the egg whites, sea salt, ground white pepper and onion powder. Place the mushroom mixture, tofu mixture and all the remaining ingredients in a bowl, and combine, using a rubber spatula.

Lightly spray a quiche pan with olive oil, pour in the frittata mixture and bake until firm – approximately 1 hour.

For the salsa sauce, spray a baking tray with oil and arrange the tomatoes, onions and shallot on it. Bake in the same oven for approximately 30 minutes. Purée the vegetables in a blender or food processor, then mix in the sea salt.

Heat the sauce in a sauté pan and sprinkle in the basil just before serving. Serve the baked frittata with the sauce spooned over.

calories per serving: 260   *fat grams per serving: 14*

chapter nine

14-Day
Carb Control Diet

Now that you have read all about the Carb Curfew diet, this chapter will show you how to start putting the diet into practice with a 24-hour-a-day strategy covering 14 days. This will allow you to see day by day how you can apply the nutritional strategies that we have discussed throughout the book. Here is a quick recap of the strategies:

- Operate the Carb Curfew – no bread, pasta, rice, potatoes or cereal after 5 p.m.
- Decrease overall fat intake – aim for no more than 40 grams of fat a day.
- Eat your fruit and vegetables – aim for five portions of fruit and vegetables a day.

- ◎ Reduce the amount of calories you consume – aim for a daily calorie intake of 1,200–1,500 calories.
- ◎ Drink two litres of water – spread evenly throughout the day.

Daily Calorie Allowance

The Carb Curfew daily calorie allowance is 1,200–1,500 calories. Here is how the calorie allowance breaks down for each meal:

breakfast: 300–350 calories
lunch: 350–400 calories
dinner: 500–550 calories
snacks: 150–200 calories (if you have a smoothie as a snack your calorie intake will be higher. Don't worry about this – as we discussed in chapter six the 80-20 rule gives you a 500 calorie cushion each day).

These are only guidelines and you don't need to stick to them rigidly. Remember, the Carb Curfew diet contains strategies which give you the flexibility to fit the diet into your lifestyle, whilst still achieving your weight-loss goals.

Carb Curfew Breakfasts

As we saw in chapter three it is important to start your day with a healthy breakfast. Here are some further suggestions for delicious breakfasts – each contains less than 350 calories.

- piece of fruit; slice of pumpernickel bread; 100g low-fat cottage cheese
- ginseng tea followed by a fruit smoothie (see below)
- 1 English muffin, split and toasted, spread thinly with quark and topped with a sliced plum
- 1 slice of wholemeal toast grilled with 25g Edam cheese and sliced tomato; small glass of orange juice
- 2 grilled tomatoes with 2 rashers grilled bacon with fat cut off; 1 slice of wholemeal toast
- 1 'skinny' American muffin with skimmed milk cappuccino

Breakfast Smoothies

As we have already seen smoothies play an important role in the Carb Curfew diet. Not only are they great as a mid-afternoon snack but they also make a delicious, filling and portable breakfast. Why not invest in a thermos flask or travelling mug so you can enjoy your smoothie when you are on the move!

Smoothies are very quick and easy to make – just follow these steps:

1. Open a small can of fruit in natural juice and pour contents into a blender.

2. Add a handful of your favourite breakfast cereal, for example, bran flakes, oatmeal, muesli, Special K or add $1/2$ tablespoon of wheatgerm.
3. Add 100g of plain or fruit low-fat yoghurt.
4. Add 200ml skimmed milk, unsweetened soya milk or skimmed goat's milk.
5. Blend and go!

Top Tip

Making your smoothie with frozen fruit will give it an extra creamy smoothness and thickness. Freeze the canned fruit on a tray – remember to separate the fruit first to make it easier to handle when frozen. Similarly, you can freeze the juice of the fruit and/or the low-fat yoghurt in an ice-cube tray and add the frozen cubes to your smoothie.

Here are some delicious fruit and cereal combos for your breakfast smoothies:

- banana with oatmeal
- apricots with malted flakes, for example, Special K
- peaches with shreddies
- prunes with bran flakes
- raspberries with wheatgerm

Carb Curfew Lunches

As we discussed in chapter three, it is really important to eat some protein in your midday meal, ideally in a ratio of one portion of starch to one portion of protein. This improves your concentration, fuels you with energy for the afternoon and helps you avoid those mid-afternoon sugar cravings. The suggestions in chapter three as well as the recipes in chapter eight provide a wide range of ideas for your midday meal. Here are some further tips and suggestions.

Sandwiches

Sandwiches are great to have at lunchtime. Open sandwiches are better than the traditional closed sandwiches as they give an excellent balance of starch and protein as well as containing fewer calories. Here are some suggestions for delicious open sandwiches – each sandwich contains less than 350 calories. To ensure you get your quota of vegetables you can pile up on the vegetable sandwich filling or munch with a cup of vegetable crudités.

Select one of the following:
- small pitta bread
- medium granary roll split in two
- small bagel, toasted
- thin slice of wholemeal bread
- small slice of focaccia bread

Pile on as many of the following as you like:

⊚ lettuce
⊚ chopped tomatoes
⊚ diced peppers
⊚ grated carrot
⊚ chopped spring onion
⊚ cucumber slices
⊚ alfalfa sprouts
⊚ beansprouts

Add a portion of one of the following:

⊚ canned tuna in brine
⊚ poached egg
⊚ chargrilled chicken breast
⊚ flavoured cottage cheese
⊚ smoked salmon
⊚ canned pink salmon
⊚ canned pilchards in tomato sauce
⊚ lean sliced smoked ham
⊚ peeled boiled prawns
⊚ grated Edam cheese

Note: See page 56 for how much a portion of starch
and protein is. As we discussed earlier, you can also visually estimate portion sizes – a portion of starch looks
roughly the same size as a portion of protein. This means
with open sandwiches you need to add a layer of protein,
such as tuna, chicken or canned salmon, approximately
the same thickness as the slice of bread or the roll.

As you cut down on the amount of fat you are consuming in the form of butter, margarine spreads and mayonnaise, you may feel that your sandwiches are dry and lacking in taste. Here are some low-fat spreads that will help keep your sandwiches moist and tasty:

- marmite
- thin scraping of quark
- fromage frais mixed with tomato salsa
- natural yoghurt mixed with a little balsamic vinegar
- grainy mustard
- reduced fat tzatziki
- tomato salsa
- fromage frais or low-fat natural yoghurt mixed with teaspoon of sweet Thai chilli sauce
- mango chutney

But remember, the Carb Curfew diet is not about cutting all fat from your diet – the essential fats are important and you can get these in sandwich toppings such as salmon and canned pilchards, and of course you can have a small amount of olive oil dressing on a side salad.

And Don't Forget About Soups

Soups can make a nourishing and filling meal at any time of the year, but as the weather gets colder soups can be a particularly satisfying, quick and portable meal. And with the extensive range of pre-prepared fresh soups (found at the chill cabinet of your supermarket) and canned soups available you really can be spoilt for choice.

Select vegetable and broth-based soups with less than 300 calories per serving. Avoid cream-based soups and always read the food labels. If you have not already got one, invest in a thermos flask so you can enjoy your soup wherever you go.

Beans or tofu are delicious added to soups and both are great sources of protein. If you are eating soup at lunchtime, serve with a portion of starch, for example, a slice of wholemeal, rye or soda bread.

Carb Curfew Dinners

As we have already discussed, the basic principle behind your Carb Curfew dinner is to omit the starches and eat instead protein (lean meat, poultry, fish, eggs and pulses) with vegetables and fruit. The recipe chapter contains some interesting ideas which you can use as treats or when having friends for supper. Or you can put the Carb Curfew into practice by simply following these guidelines. Select one protein food from the following list:

- ◎ 150g lean meat, all visible fat cut off, or poultry
- ◎ 150g white fish or shellfish, for example, cod, peeled prawns, plaice

- 100g oily fish, for example, mackerel, salmon, tuna, herring, pilchards
- 2 eggs
- 150g cooked pulses, for example, kidney beans, lentils, chick peas, haricot beans

Avoid high fat content meats such as sausages and trim fat off meat before cooking.

Serve with unlimited vegetables. This list will give you some ideas: cabbage, carrots, peas, cauliflower, lettuce, spinach, tomatoes, watercress, fennel, courgettes, leeks, brussels sprouts, broccoli, runner beans, bean sprouts, water chestnuts, sweetcorn, mushrooms, broad beans, onions, peppers, marrow, pumpkin, turnip, to name just a few.

Select one of the following cooking methods:

- braise
- steam
- bake
- microwave
- boil
- dry roast
- casserole
- grill
- poach

Avoid frying and watch out for stir-frying and sautéing as this can add an enormous amount of fat and calories. Do not add additional fat or oils to vegetables.

Sweet tooth? Finish your meal with fresh fruit, a low-fat yoghurt or fruit sorbet.

Daily Allowance

Each day you must have:

- ◉ Half a pint of skimmed or semi-skimmed milk or 150g pot of low-fat yoghurt
- ◉ No more than two cups of tea or coffee a day
- ◉ Two litres of water spread evenly throughout the day
- ◉ Five portions of fruit and vegetables

14-Day Carb Control Diet

Day 1

Breakfast: porridge made with ½ teacup of porridge oats and 1 teacup of milk, topped with 1 chopped apple; small glass freshly squeezed orange juice

Lunch: Smoked Chicken and Mexican Black Bean Salad (see recipe on page 162) served with slice of granary bread; slice of melon

Dinner: Carb Curfew main course* served with salad or vegetables of your choice; small bowl of fruit sorbet

Optional snacks: can of tomato juice; 150g pot low-fat fruit yoghurt

Day 2

Breakfast: 1 teacup of Special K with skimmed milk from allowance and handful of raspberries; small glass of orange juice

Lunch: any carton of fresh vegetable soup under 300 calories – add ½ cup kidney beans and serve with 2 crispbreads; 1 pear

Dinner: Carb Curfew main course* served with salad or vegetables of your choice; small bowl stewed fruit

Optional snacks: 1 apple; 150g pot low-fat fruit yoghurt

Day 3

Breakfast: ½ grapefruit with teaspoon sugar; porridge made with milk (same as day 1)

Lunch: open sandwich with meat, fish or cheese (under 350 calories), served with small bag of vegetable crudités with salsa; 1 apple

Dinner: Carb Curfew main course* served with salad or vegetables of your choice; slice of pineapple

Optional snacks: small glass orange juice; 1 kiwi fruit

Day 4

Breakfast: large bowl of fresh fruit salad; 1 slice wholemeal toast spread with a thin layer of quark and reduced sugar jam

Lunch: medium-size jacket potato topped with small pot of low-fat cottage cheese and served with small green salad; small glass of orange or apple juice

Dinner: Carb Curfew main course* served with salad or vegetables of your choice; small bowl stewed fruit

Optional snacks: banana smoothie; 1 apple

Day 5

Breakfast: porridge made with water, add a handful of chopped apple and serve with 2 tablespoons of natural yoghurt

Lunch: open sandwich with meat, fish or cheese (under 350 calories); small glass of orange juice or apple juice

Dinner: Carb Curfew main course* served with salad or vegetables of your choice; small bowl of fruit sorbet

Optional snacks: 1 kiwi fruit; 1 pear

Day 6

Breakfast: $1/2$ grapefruit with $1/2$ teaspoon of sugar; 1 slice wholemeal toast with marmite and cottage cheese

Lunch: Vegetables Menestra (see recipe page 161); 150g pot low-fat fruit yoghurt

Dinner: Carb Curfew main course* served with salad or vegetables of your choice; 1 banana

Optional snacks: can of vegetable juice; 1 orange

Day 7

Breakfast: large bowl of fresh fruit salad; 2 Ryvita with thin scraping of quark and topped with sliced plum

Lunch: poached egg with 1 toasted bagel; small glass of orange or apple juice
Dinner: Carb Curfew main course* served with salad or vegetables of your choice; small bowl fruit sorbet
Optional snacks: 150g pot natural bio yoghurt with 1 teaspoon honey; 1 kiwi fruit

Day 8

Breakfast: porridge made with water and served with 2 tablespoons natural bio yoghurt and 1 chopped apple; small glass freshly squeezed orange juice
Lunch: mixed medium sushi box (250g); small glass apple or orange juice
Dinner: Carb Curfew main course* served with salad or vegetables of your choice; 150g pot low-fat fruit fromage frais
Optional snacks: cup of grapes; 1 can vegetable juice

Day 9

Breakfast: large bowl of fresh fruit salad with 150g pot low-fat bio yoghurt
Lunch: Mexican-style Wrap with Beans, Herbs and Vegetables (see recipe on page 160); low-fat chocolate mousse
Dinner: Carb Curfew main course* served with salad or vegetables of your choice; small bowl of fruit sorbet
Optional snacks: 300ml shop-bought fruit smoothie; 1 banana

Day 10

Breakfast: Swiss muesli made with $1/2$ cup porridge oats soaked overnight with milk from allowance and 1 teacup of water, mixed with small handful of sultanas, a grated apple and a pinch of nutmeg

Lunch: homemade chef salad made with 28g lean chicken breast, 28g lean ham, 56g cottage cheese, lettuce, tomatoes, onion, cucumber and peppers; serve with 1 slice rye bread; 1 pear

Dinner: Carb Curfew main course* served with salad or vegetables of your choice; small bowl stewed fruit

Optional snacks: 1 kiwi fruit; 1 can vegetable juice

Day 11

Breakfast: 1 cup bran flakes cereal with skimmed milk from allowance and small banana

Lunch: 1 medium jacket potato with 150g pot cottage cheese with chopped tomato and fresh basil; serve with a side salad or bag of vegetable sticks; small glass of orange or apple juice

Dinner: Carb Curfew main course served with salad or vegetables of your choice; slice of melon

Optional snacks: 1 cup seedless grapes; 150g pot low-fat bio yoghurt

Day 12

Breakfast: Swiss muesli with sultanas and grated apple (same as day 10)

Lunch: 1 slice wholemeal toast with small can baked beans and 2 grilled tomatoes; small glass of orange or apple juice

Dinner: Carb Curfew main course* served with salad or vegetables of your choice; small bowl of pineapple in natural juice

Optional snacks: 150g pot low-fat bio yoghurt; slice of melon

Day 13

Breakfast: large fresh fruit salad with 150g pot natural low-fat bio yoghurt

Lunch: toasted bagel with 2 slices smoked trout or salmon, served with green salad; slice of melon

Dinner: Carb Curfew main course* served with salad or vegetables of your choice; low-fat chocolate mousse

Optional snacks: 1 small banana; small glass of orange or apple juice

Day 14

Breakfast: 1 poached egg on 1 slice dry wholemeal toast; small glass orange juice

Lunch: medium-size jacket potato with small can of tuna in brine and small green salad; 1 pear

Dinner: Carb Curfew main course* served with salad or vegetables of your choice; small bowl of fruit sorbet

Optional snacks: 1 apple; 150g pot low-fat bio yoghurt

* Choose any of the Carb Curfew dinner recipes from the Carb Curfew Recipes chapter or create your own main course using the Carb Curfew guidelines discussed earlier.

Index